Doctors learn more from their patients than from formal lectures in medical school. Diane Jepsen has taught generations of young doctors about brain lymphoma. She has the skill to cope with her illness, conquer it and then step outside to see it in perspective. She is a model for others and a survivor.

Fred H. Hochberg, M.D.
Neuro-oncologist
Massachusetts General Hospital
Boston, Massachusetts

Although every person who has a serious neurological problem has their own unique story, Diane's compelling narrative is a special source of both amazement and inspiration. Afflicted as she was in the prime of her life with a cerebellum lymphoma, she has not only survived but thrived through years of onerous treatment. The very survival is itself a marvel, but it is her invincible courage of spirit that is an inspiration to all who know her. As she herself once said, "Don't worry Dr. Moore, I'm Fadel tough."

Michael J. Moore, M.D., P.C.
Neurological Medicine
Emerson Hospital
Concord, Massachusetts

The story of a woman whose illness made her feel and act like a baby all over again is a reminder to the rest of us that our lives and livelihoods hang by a slender thread. Often when we meet adversity, we conclude that the thread is severed and cannot be reunited. But, Diane, like an ingenious spider, respun the thread of her vitality and reconnected to her family and friends.

To her physician, Diane's journey from helplessness to control comes as no surprise. She has always had the gift of lighting candles—not cursing the darkness. To me, the delight is her willingness to share her extraordinary experience, so private, yet so universal, with the world.

Henry W. Vaillant, M.D., Internist
Acton Medical Associates, P.C.
Acton, Massachusetts

In *Last Trip to Baker 5,* Diane Jepsen takes us along for the ride. The terrain is her journey, battle and ultimate victory in fighting brain cancer. With her humor and candid prose, she recounts the highs and lows of her challenges and lets the reader know how to fight life's battles and win.

Of all the individuals profiled in my book on coping with concealed chronic illness, Diane Jepsen's story was most inspirational and her strength was spectacular to behold.

> Carol Sveilich, M.A.
> Author of *Just Fine: Unmasking Concealed Chronic Illness and Pain*
> San Diego, California

Diane Jepsen's amazing true-life journey through the diagnosis, treatment and healing of brain lymphoma provides both an inspiring and informative message of value and interest to people of all ages. The power of her spirit and never-give-up attitude combined with the top medical treatment and guidance, gives hope to anyone facing life challenges. A must read that is life changing.

> Kelly Ferrin, Gerontologist
> Author of *What's Age Got to Do With it?*
> San Diego, California

LAST TRIP TO BAKER 5

LAST TRIP TO BAKER 5

BEATING BRAIN CANCER TWICE

Diane Fadel Jepsen

Writer's Showcase

New York Lincoln Shanghai

Last Trip to Baker 5
Beating Brain Cancer Twice

Writer's Showcase
an imprint of iUniverse, Inc.

iUniverse books may be ordered through booksellers or by contacting:

iUniverse
2021 Pine Lake Road, Suite 100
Lincoln, NE 68512
www.iuniverse.com
1-800-Authors (1-800-288-4677)

Third Edition

ISBN-13: 978-0-595-21880-6
ISBN-13: 0-595-21880-6

Printed in the United States of America

DEDICATION

Following is a remarkable story of one woman's experience with brain cancer, not once, but twice. It tells the struggle of a seemingly unending battle with a long list of soldiers. The generals of these two battles were my brave and courageous mother, Alice Christie (Paolina), and my saint of a sister, Georgia Tamoush, who were my lifelines. I thank them from the bottom of my heart and my entire body and soul. God sent them to me about a half century ago, but recently I completely felt their love, and realized their unfailing strength and endurance.

Thank you Mom, for believing in me, encouraging me with your patience and your positive attitude, which was reflected unknowingly back to me. Thank you for staying calm by my side, and never giving up. Thank you for knowing when to lend me a hand, and knowing when to let go, allowing me to develop independence. Thank you for your everlasting love.

Thank you, Georgia, for working through all the details to make this story as accurate as possible, as I could not remember some conversations, and I was not present when others took place. You have an extraordinary sense of space and recall, and I would not have been able to do this without you. Actually, I would not be living to write this without you continually, loving me by my side. You are an incredible human being, and you are the miracle, not I!

I heartily dedicate this book to both of you.

CONTENTS

FOREWORD

by Dr. Henry Vaillant

What a pleasure and honor it is to introduce this book. Diane Jepsen undertook this project during the early phase of her convalescence at a time when she could scarcely sign her name. This account of her fast-forward recovery speaks for itself. Her honesty and tenacity inspire all of us: fellow cancer victims, ordinary people, and those caregivers who have devoted their lives to helping those like her.

A number of things stand out in this work, first and foremost is the unquenchable spirit of the author herself. Undaunted by an illness that felled her in the prime of her life, she always kept her priorities straight. First was her own health and self-knowledge. She went to bed at night with weights on her bed, so she could awaken to her exhausting exercise program each morning. "Whatever happens, you'll be able to handle it because you are a strong woman," said her 87-year-old roommate during her first hospitalization. Truer words were never spoken. The inner light and discipline that distinguish Diane remained even in moments of despair. Where many might lapse into sorrowful self-absorption, she never lost sight of her parenting responsibility. Even when she could only crawl, she reminded her two sons to pick up their socks. Even when she had a needle taped to her arm vein, she visited a dying friend.

The story of a woman whose illness made her feel and act like a baby all over again is a reminder to the rest of us that our lives and livelihoods hang by a slender thread. Often when we meet adversity, we conclude that the thread is severed and cannot be reunited. But Diane, like an ingenious spider, re-spun the thread of her vitality and reconnected to her family and friends. "I am going to make it through this. I have a lot more living to do," she told us—and so she has.

Her journal is simply stated. The only Boswell we meet here is her faithful dog. The only cancer ward is Baker 5, and Diane has eyes only for the kindness of the people she meets there. But, the power in this document is not merely literary; it is the ongoing human struggle to survive and live meaningfully. From the horror of being trapped in a carwash, to the warmth of her first dance, from the time she donned her panties standing up, to her first haircut after the ordeal, the reader is alongside of her cheering her on. Diane complains that her handwriting is blurry, but the incandescent spirit behind her words shines through, just as brightly as the spotlight she once danced in.

To her physician, Diane's journey from helplessness to control comes as no surprise. She has always had the gift of lighting candles—not cursing the darkness. To me, the delight is her willingness to share her extraordinary experience, so private, and yet so universal, with the world. Diane, as she says herself, is "a good teacher...sensitive to others and aware of their needs." She has touched us all with what she quaintly terms a "phantom hand." Let us respond in kind.

PREFACE

The purpose of this book is twofold: First, I wanted to write about my experience in dealing with a rare brain cancer, Cerebellum Lymphoma. I needed to document my trials and victories, partly as therapy, partly so I could put everything behind me. In addition, the book would function as a mirror of my feelings, and a record of my progress. Secondly, I hope this will be a help and an inspiration to other cancer patients and their families and friends, or anyone else facing seemingly impossible odds, or frustrations.

ACKNOWLEDGEMENTS

My deep gratitude and heartfelt thanks to the following:

My mother, Alice Fadel Christie (presently, Alice Christie Paolina) and her husband, Dean now deceased; my brother, Jim Fadel and wife Arleen and my sisters Georgia Tamoush and husband Ron and Linda Willey; my children, Peter and David Jepsen; my deceased father, George Fadel, for being a model of strength and integrity; my former mother-in-law and friend, Esther Jepsen; Drs.Vaillant, Hochberg, Moore, Cantu, Pruitt, Gibai, Smith, Hayes, Levine, Lingood, Vinger, Lessell, Newman, and others too numerous to mention; my therapists, Jane Loureiro, Pat White, Kathy Warren, Sue Beverage; Pam Sawyer of Acton Public Nursing Service; Lorna Harris, nurse at Acton Medical Associates, all the nurses and technicians at Emerson Hospital, Concord, Massachusetts (especially intensive care); Massachusetts General Hospital, Boston, Massachusetts; Waltham Hospital, Massachusetts; and Rina Spence, President of Emerson Hospital.

Aubrey Mackall, Donna Graceffa, Judy Burgess, Valerie Carlson, Kay Costello, Ellen Valade, Joyce Johnson, Molly Klau, Nancy Nephew, Lynn Porter, Linda Sarles, Ann Melia, John Moniz, Karl Karash, other friends at GenRad, and Fran Portante.

Peg Snook. Ray and Caroline Tripp, Lynn Hughes, Fran Harris, Fatina Kerr, Elizabeth Warren, Jo Small, Betty Gooding, Sally Blute, Valerie Spotkill, Patti Vega, Sara James, Betsy Dickerman, Gretchen Olenberger, Jan Stearns, Carol Kuenzler, Ann and Dick Hosmer, Betty Oliver, Madeline Kadaboski, Carol Aaron, Claire Abare, Sandy Hall, Peg Reedy, Paula Kwon, Barbara Lauritzen, and friends at Theatre III. Also, Robin Wurster, Judy Shaffer, Bev Seward, Mary Lou Paradise, Kathy O'Grady, Karen Murray, Michael Lemere, Maureen Chicella, Petra, Tina Close, Linda and Ed Vitiello, Jane Johnson, Peg Hittner, a housekeeper/helper who wanted to be mentioned as "George." Johanna Menezes, Kathy Sheehan, Rita Sharkey, Anita Coffey, Maggie Vassilopoulos, Bernie Reynolds, Peter Dolan (yoga guru instructor), Cindy Armstrong, Joan Batman, Amy and Jennifer Griffith, Elaine Romeo, Adelle Little, Jackie Mapletoft, Mary Beth Quigley, friends of Minuteman Ridge; Muxie; and my little friends, Rachel Valade, Theresa Portante, and Shawn Melia; Judy York's third grade class at St. Bridget's School: Kate, Meghan, Steve, Garrett, Bobby and Bill; Jim Potter, friend and technical support; Billy Irwin, proofreader and support; Bob Weber, and all who sent get well wishes and prayers, coast to coast, and around the world; and finally, my dog, Boswell, for sticking extra close by.

1.

THE BEGINNING OF A NIGHTMARE

Nineteen eighty seven was the worst year of my life. No matter what, I will never have another year like that one. I'm not sure when this all started. In retrospect, why did I have so many headaches with nausea? Probably migraines. I'll try "Benson's Relaxation Response." Why did I get so sick at the restaurant or on the plane that time? Maybe it was because, when I was in my twenties, I was in a car accident, and got a big lump on my head. I was doing all the right things: I did yoga. I ate well. I didn't drink or smoke. Maybe I was born this way. Maybe there was a little cancer cell somewhere. I look back and guess when everything started to happen. Not one human being on this earth knows. Not any doctors, or scientists or even psychics.

I started to feel really badly in January. I was told I had a severe case of labyrinthitis (inflammation in the ear resulting in vertigo). My CAT Scan showed nothing, but I knew something was wrong. I was dizzy and my vision was blurry. Objects would just sort of move around. I missed about two-and-a-half months of work, went back half days, and then was laid off. I was told by my manager they had to reduce their sales department (I was the sales coordinator.), even at their branches in California. I was sort of glad because I was so sick. I tried everything at this point. Meclizine. Why did it work on my friend, but not on me? I tried the patch behind the ear. I then decided to see an

1

acupuncturist and a nutritionist. I progressively got better, and in May and most of June, I was feeling top-notch. Walking three to four miles a day. Doing 20 full pushups. Feeling very fit.

I helped take care of a good friend who was suffering from cancer. I would do errands for her, make lunch and milkshakes, and just spend some time with her. I started feeling dizzy and nauseous again when I took my friend shopping in Boston. One of her friends was closing her designer's clothing shop, and we were going in to get some good deals. I noticed I was getting dizzy reaching up to get the clothes to try them on. She felt weak and so did I, but we both came out of there with a bundle. I never mentioned anything to her about my weakened condition.

I took her to radiation, and helped her choose a wig. In a few months, she lost her battle. Little did I know I would be revisiting the same hospital, the same waiting room, the same radiation nurse, etc.

The last week in June I was feeling very badly, dizzy again, vomiting, not able to eat. I was told that I may have a reoccurrence of labyrinthitis, but I didn't think it would happen this soon. My son, David, had an early birthday party on June 23, and I remember struggling through that!

By July 4th, I was too sick to even care about fireworks. My brother, Jim, from California, knew even by phone, that perhaps I wasn't getting enough nutrition, and suggested we get some balanced frozen dinners. At least I would be getting food from all the groups. My mother, also from California, knew something was wrong. I tried to reassure her that I would get better, but I never did.

2.

THE MS SCARE

Not long after that, I was literally crawling to the shower. I had just washed my hair and put on a fresh nightgown. I remember which one. Cotton. Lavender on the bottom and a white fitted bodice. My mother gave it to me. Said it looked like me.

Aubrey, my friend, had come to visit. He brought me some pink carnations. I was so sick with nausea and vomiting. At that point, my friend, Donna, happened to call, heard me on the phone, and said she thought I should go to the hospital. She arrived in no time flat. Aubrey carried me down the steps—nightgown and bare feet. Donna got in the driver's seat of her car. I just remember telling Aubrey to be careful. I don't know how he carried me down the steps. He is a large man and a strong man, but I have always felt "heavy." I thought his feet would slip off the steps, and then we would both fall.

I distinctly remember Aubrey carrying me out the front door. I also remember the pounding of his feet on the ground, as he took each step. I still don't know how he managed to slip me into the back seat of the car. He sat next to me, holding me, as I held a paper bag. It was early in the evening, and it was misty and foggy. It was a silent ride to Emerson Hospital. I was sick, and my friends were scared. Donna didn't waste any time getting there.

Emergency room first. Checked vital signs. Gave me an IV of glucose water. The doctor said I could either leave in a couple hours, or spend the night. I knew I had to stay, and my friends were very angry the doctor would even think of sending me home. They never would have allowed me to go anyway.

I was finally put in a quad room. I had an 87-year-old roommate who was having hip surgery. She had difficulty remembering where she was most of the time. Pretty soon two more patients came in. Another elderly woman was up from cardiac care, and she had many visitors. It sounded like a garden party around her all the time. The woman next to me was having elective surgery, and was coughing all the time. My first roommate always had her TV on. I particularly remember the Red Sox playing. Everything was too noisy; everything bothered me. The "garden party" woman was released. Good news for her, I remember. I was feeling more dependent as time went on. I couldn't walk to the bathroom without a nurse.

The location of the call button on my bed got to be the most important thing to me. I was too sick to be moving around to look for it. Still feeling nauseous and vomiting all the time. Many times the other women would awaken me, because either one couldn't find her call button, or the other was coughing too hard to locate hers. I *always* knew where my button was.

I had different neurological tests. This is when I met Dr. Moore. He seemed very knowledgeable. He was tall, wore reading glasses, seemed British. My friends and I secretly referred to him as "Icabod," the name I gave him. I heard him administering some of the same tests on patients in nearby rooms, as he did on me.

A hospital social worker came to talk to me about my fears, and tried to prepare me for what might happen. She gave me a paper on loss and grief, which I threw aside. First of all, the print was too small and poorly printed for me to see. Secondly, I wasn't in the mood to read about that anyway! I just knew that before I got sick, I was doing 20 full pushups a day, and now I would have to start from peg one. My primary doctor, Dr. Vaillant, said he set up some home services for me, just in case. I thought, "Uh-oh."

I was finally ordered to have an MRI (Magnetic Resonance Imaging) test. The ambulance personnel came into my room with a stretcher, unexpectedly on time. One of them yelled out, "Diane Jepsen!"

I called out from behind my curtain, "She went home!" Once again I resigned myself to a no-choice situation, and decided I would, at least, enjoy my ambulance ride. I felt good being hoisted up; some of those women are really strong! I did a lot of chatting and a lot of looking around the inside. I had never been in an ambulance before, so I wanted to enjoy it, and make the best of it. Sounds kind of weird, but that's how I felt.

No matter what anyone else says, the MRI test was definitely one of the worst experiences of my life. In a documentary on TV, they showed a woman taking the test; they were showing how painless and effortless it was. They made it look easy and quite pleasant. I have another friend who said he slept two hours during his test. Let's put it this way. If you're the least bit claustrophobic, it's not a day at the beach! My doctor gave me some Valium, but when it was time for the test, I was not relaxed. I said to myself, "Here I have to go into that thing, and I am not relaxed! And what if I have to vomit?" They slide your whole body into a big tube, and tell you that you will hear some loud banging noises, which will get continually louder, and that if you want to come out, you can't go back in again.

Well, I wanted the test to be right, and I always wanted to be tough and cooperate, so I called on all my resources. Knowing that it wouldn't last forever, probably about an hour, was a saving grace. (That's how I feel about having a tooth drilled at the dentist. Taking novocaine is worse than a few minutes of drilling, so I don't take it. Instead, I roll my eyes back and think of something else, something pleasant.) First, I said a prayer. I knew that God wouldn't give me more than I could handle. I did some deep "yoga" breathing, and thought about my Club Med vacations. This thought came to me: One should stay mentally and physically and spiritually strong, because you never know when you'll need to call upon those resources.

What my 87-year-old roommate said, kept resounding in my head:

"What's there is there. And whatever happens, you will be able to handle it, because you are a strong woman."

That evening Dr. V. said that four pairs of eyes looked at the X-rays, and there was no sign of a major tumor. I was relieved. No tumor was showing up.

In the next morning or two, I was to find out the actual results/diagnosis. Also, my brother, Jim, not knowing what he was about ready to learn, arrived just in time to hear the doctor give me the diagnosis. Or, maybe he waited for my brother to arrive so he *could* tell me. When he told us I had Multiple Sclerosis, I started to cry. Jim was in shock, but he was very consoling. I don't know what I would have done without him. He talked to the doctor, and proceeded to order me a cane from physical therapy. When the therapist brought the canes, I wanted to throw them against the wall. I knew I had to accept it, but I felt even worse for my mom. My older sister has Multiple Sclerosis.

So, we went home. I wobbled into the house, and on the kitchen counter was a cake that my younger son, David, had baked. It said "Get Well Soon." My heart sank. I had to tell both kids I had Multiple Sclerosis. I can still see David kneeling on my bed, as he cried and said, "Are you going to die?" (As I am typing this, I am crying, thinking of his head thrown back, and his face in tears.) I said, "I'm not going to die. I have to go to your basketball games!" Peter stoically said, "You'll get better. You were sick and got better before, and you'll do it again." (referring to the labyrinthitis diagnosis)

Jim got stuck taking care of me and the kids. I was almost totally helpless, and the kids had their activities, and had to be driven places. He made unbelievably great meals, took care of the bills and any arriving mail, and had to deal with all my neighbors and friends, which turned out to be overwhelming! He tried to get me to walk with my cane from the light switch to my bed (few yards). I wanted to do it, and tried hard, but I was so sick. Nausea and vomiting. I forced myself to do a few pushups. I figured if I could still do that, I would be okay. But, I got even worse.

After about a week or more, my brother left. He precooked meals, so we could eat well for a few days, when my mother would arrive. She stayed about a month, did a lot of nurturing and a lot of cooking. I slept downstairs on the couch. It was getting hot and I needed the air conditioner in the family room. Also, it was too hard to climb the steps to my bedroom.

I had to have the ACTH IV treatment at home for 13 days, eight hours a day. I had a heparin lock that had to be changed every two to three days. A visiting nurse came to the house, and showed my mother and me exactly what to do. My friend, Donna, was there and took notes for us "Put alcohol on everything, and don't let anything touch the ground. When the alarm sounds, look to see what the problem is. The message will say OCCLUSION or something else. If there is a problem, call us any time, day or night (which I did)."

Sometimes my mom and I were up in the middle of the night, trying to figure out a problem. I had to eat with the IV pole by my side, and take it to the bathroom with me. A couple of times in the middle of the night, I had to urinate in a big pink plastic wash basin. Mom stayed cool, so I stayed cool.

It was about this time that my friend, Jane, was dying in the hospital. We had been talking on the phone, when she was still able to do that. I very much resented not being able to be with her. Her daughters called me when she was nearing the end. I called a store and asked them to describe their stuffed animals to me. Then I sent a friend to pick up the white stuffed cat I had just chosen over the phone. (I thought that maybe my dying friend might be able to feel something soft.)

At 1 a.m. I was thinking about her and wrote the following poem in five minutes: (I had a very hard time sleeping anyway because of the medication.)

To my dear friend, Jane—a woman of grace, beauty and intelligence. You are a miracle.

> A soul
> Entrapped in a body
> Eager to go
> From a cavern of pain
> To a land of Love;
> Let your spirit fly
> And leave your earthly temple;
> Meet your Maker;
> Bon Voyage;
> It's see you later,
> But not goodbye.
>
> Love,
> Diane

I then had another friend take it to the framer. Next, I took the cat and framed poem to her hospital room. I was transported in a wheelchair by a volunteer up to Jane's room. I still had the heparin-lock for my IV in my arm. I don't know if she knew I was there, but I still talked to her and told her that I loved her. I went to her wake and her funeral. I was still in the middle of treatments, and Mom was worried about me. She suggested I go to the wake or the funeral, but I did both.

Michael, my friend and dancing partner from Theatre III, the community theater one mile from my house, came to visit. Before he came, he asked on the phone, "What do you want me to bring you?" I said, "Something soft." He brought me a little stuffed bunny, a "get-well bunny," that had been passed around several times. He has MS, and someone gave him this bunny, to give to someone else when he felt well. So, when I started to feel better, I passed it on to a mother of one of my son's friends, who was in a bad car accident.

I wanted to be well informed of my situation, so people brought me all kinds of information on MS. I became very upset and cried, so my mother took everything away from me.

After a month, I told her she should leave, that this MS disease is an up and down thing, and that I would be fine. I was feeling a little better after the treatment, and my friends would help out. I was told that I should expect to experience a "downer" or the "blahs" after the treatment, which I did. But, on top of all that, I kept getting worse. It took more effort to speak. My coordination was worsening. Nausea and vomiting. Vision more blurred.

3.

THE TUMOR

Dr. Vaillant, my primary care doctor, was visiting in Africa, so I went to see another doctor, and then on to Dr. Moore, my neurologist. Aubrey and my next-door neighbor, Linda, took me. I was transported by wheelchair from the car to the office, and I was vomiting and couldn't hold my head up. I remember Aubrey lifting me up onto the examining table. The next thing I heard was Dr. Moore instructing someone to take me to intensive care. Then I knew I must *really* be sick!

First, I had to be admitted through Emergency. (I had been here not too long ago.) Soon after admission, I had a CAT Scan. The tumor *finally* showed up! The next day, August 26, I remember Drs. Moore and Cantu, the brain surgeon, standing at the foot of my bed. They started poking and prodding me. Aubrey was there and heard the phrases, "life-threatening" and "marked deterioration." The pressure in my head was building up. They asked if they could take a biopsy of my brain. What does one say to that?!! Like maybe, do I have a few weeks to think this over? I said, "I am too confused to think."

I don't know how I remembered my mother's telephone number in California. And I don't know how she happened to hear the phone; she was outside in the very back part of her yard. What would have happened if she were not home, or did not hear the phone? Just lucky, I guess!

I could hear Dr. Moore talking to her at the nurses' station. "We have a very sick girl here." He brought the phone into my room. (I had room No.1, the most intensive care room in the unit.) Mom pleasantly said to me, "Honey, I think you should go ahead, and I'll be there when you wake up." In retrospect, I don't know how she managed to keep her composure on the phone.

The phone was taken from me. I was immediately put on a stretcher, and taken to the operating room. Before I was taken, I said to Dr. Cantu, "I hear you are a very good surgeon." I figured I should get on his good side from the beginning!

The last thing I remember was being in the operating room, and having the anesthetist and others scurrying about, doing their business. It amazed me that that is exactly what it was. They were very calm. I just remember the mask, and after that, nothing. I was finally returned to intensive care with tubes everywhere and a bag of something soft—my hair! I was told they have to give you your hair for legal reasons!!

I heard my mother's voice in the hall. It was a wonderful secure feeling, knowing she was there with me. Little did I know the trauma she must have been going through, and the little things she had to do to get ready for an indefinite stay. Coming from different locations in California, she and Georgia, my sister, and Jim, my brother, came on the same cramped flight. After a long uncomfortable flight, they went straight to the hospital from the airport! Thank God, they were all there!

They were all so cool with the doctors (I had a lot of them.), and asked informative questions, as they muddled through all the mysteries which were still vague to the doctors. They all were at the hospital early each morning to talk to the doctors. They were concerned. They were smart. I am so proud to belong to this family. Loving teamwork—that's one way I'd describe it. I am sure I was not totally aware of the late hours they spent discussing this tragedy.

The tumor was malignant. Now let's see—is the cancer anywhere else? At this point, I didn't care. Bone marrow test. Liver and spleen. The thoracic region. The whole body. My family anxiously awaited the results, but I didn't care. I never asked one question about a test result. I didn't care, and I guess I just didn't want to hear it.

I hated taking the tests. It was an inconvenience and a bother. It was hard for me to get up and be transferred to the stretcher. Plus, it seemed I always had to wait before a test and after a test, before I was transported back to my bed. This waiting was very tiring and hard for me. Ironically, I used to work as a hospital volunteer at this hospital in the transport department, and now I was the one being transported. Being transported is a real dependence and a real loss of control.

I remember before one test, Georgia was feeding me the required liquid through a straw. I had to drink four big glasses. I will never forget how good she was, how understanding, how tender. She said, "You only have a little bit more to go, because the glass is bigger at the top." You can't imagine how a simple comment such as that brought me relief.

Intensive care at Emerson Hospital has the best, most compassionate nurses in the country, I am sure. In one sense, I really hated being there, because the only control you have is your call button. No TV (wasn't interested anyway.), no phone, no button to control head and foot levels of the mattress, no bathroom (couldn't use one anyway).

Immediately after my surgery, I started my period, and I couldn't take care of myself. I felt like a baby. I *was* a baby.

I always wondered how people got to a point where they didn't want to live. What is the tolerance level? If they would have given me the choice of taking "the black pill," I would have taken it. I couldn't stand. My right leg and foot turned in, so I was listing to the right. Not long ago, I was dancing on the stage, and now I couldn't even stand up. The right side of my face was drooping and was numb, as with novocaine. Even the right side of my tongue. (Later I chewed bubble gum a lot to try to help.) My vision was not only doubled, but crossed. The hearing in my right ear was muffled. Like a two-month-old infant, I could not turn over. I slobbered. It took so much energy to laugh, to talk, to swallow, to breathe. I had made out my will. The kids were well taken care of, and I certainly did not want to go on.

A of couple times the kids came to see me. I remember I really didn't want them to see me so sick, with tubes everywhere. At one point, I tried making a lesson out of it, and talked to them about the various tubes and their uses— the oxygen tube, the urine catheter, etc. Peter was 16 years old at this time; David, 13. I remember David lifting his foot and showing me his new sneakers. School was about ready to begin.

I remember being awakened in the middle of the night to answer some "memory" questions. "Where are you?" "What is your name?" "What month is it?" I said, "I don't know what month it is. It is raining outside, and school is about ready to start. It must be February. "Well, obviously, it was September, and not February. I had flunked the test!

I also remembered having to wear inflatable stockings to keep the circulation going, and to prevent blood clots. I hated that so much, and soon I had talked them into letting me take them off. I said I would exercise my legs by pushing them against the back of the bed.

Only family was to come into intensive care to visit, but my close friends, and even some not so very close friends, slipped in. Five church people came in, three with white collars. I thought I was having my last rites! Some people who couldn't come to visit sent their church leaders. Other doctors came in, including Dr. Vinger, an ophthalmologist, and Dr. Tripp, the kids' pediatrician. Dr. Tripp was so kind and so sensitive, and said, "Let me know if I can talk to the kids, or if they become too clingy." (Then he gave me a kiss on the cheek.) They never did. They never missed a beat.

Soon I was begging Drs. Moore and Cantu to let me go upstairs. I was "being good;" I was eating well. Taking my liquids. Vital signs good. I wanted to take that next step. I was taking Decadron, a steroid, to help cut down the swelling in the brain. They had to remove as much of the tumor as they could, and actually had to remove a piece of bone. I get the "heebie-geebies" when I think they had to remove part of my brain! All I could think of was the character who had a lobotomy in *One Flew Over the Cuckoo's Nest!*

Upstairs now. Private room. Nice room. Not as much attention as in intensive care, of course, but more control. I had buttons to adjust the height of my bed, and the angle of my head and my feet. TV. Telephone. More control. More visitors. David brought me a banner that said "Get Well Soon," about 10 times, which was hung in the room around the bulletin board. Later, I took that home, and had it taped to the beam in my family room. I tested the double vision of my eyes every day on it. Two banners or one? It finally came out to be one on the left side, and angled out to two, becoming more obtuse on the far right side (the most affected side of my body).

More tests. I particularly remember the bone marrow at this time. I was kidding around saying that they just put me in a remote room, because I might be screaming with pain. There were three people. I jokingly asked if they had taken this test, so they would know what their patients had to go through. A lot of fast-talking and a sense of humor got me through almost everything; plus my other resources, as I have mentioned before.

After about a week and many bouquets of flowers and cards and stuffed animals (particularly a huge teddy bear that I hauled everywhere, even to Mass

General), I was finally on my way home. Little did I know this was just the beginning of a long journey.

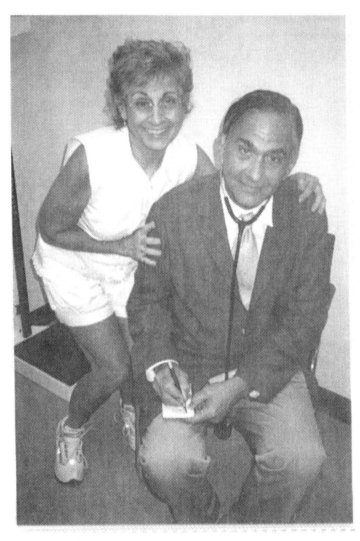

Diane Fadel Jepsen and Dr. Fred Hochberg
August 2, 2004
Massachusetts General Hospital
Cox Building, Suite 315
Boston, Massachusetts

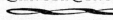

MASSACHUSETTS GENERAL HOSPITAL
CANCER CENTER™

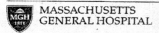

MASSACHUSETTS GENERAL HOSPITAL

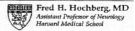

Fred H. Hochberg, MD
Assistant Professor of Neurology
Harvard Medical School

Stephen E. And Catherine Pappas Center for Neuro-Oncology
55 Fruit Street, Cox 315
Boston, Massachusetts 02114
Tel: 617 724-8770, Fax: 617 724-8769

Email: fhochberg@partners.org
November 10, 2004

Diane Jepsen
4739 Majorca Way
Oceanside, CA 92056

Dear Diane:

I have known you for 17 years. Your continued triumphs over the initial malignant brain lymphoma tell a story of the evolution of our thinking about this disease during the last 20 years. Your courage in the face of your illness tells a story of the triumph of strength and conviction in the face of cancer.

When I first met you, the illness of brain lymphoma was an incurable rare disease. Indeed in the 50 years before the early 1980's fewer than 1 patient each year was seen at the Massachusetts General Hospital bearing the diagnosis of brain lymphoma. The illness then was treated as a rarity, patients were provided with radiation therapy, very few of them survived.

Your treatment of the brain lymphoma in the 1990's with methotrexate based chemotherapy mirrored our increased understanding at that time of the role of drug therapy in comparison to radiation. Your strength during this time was an important factor for all of us who took care of you.

We now understand brain lymphoma to involve the eye, the spinal fluid, and the nerves. We are increasingly aware of the reason why these tumor cells spread to the nervous system. The body clearly has a mechanism for destroying the tumor in all organs except for the brain and we would hope to take advantage of this mechanism to see that the brain lesions also respond.

Doctors can learn from patients. We have learned from you the strength of the will to survive, the ability to deal with adversity, and the never ending sense that there lies the possibility of cure. As I have known you I have also experienced your triumphs, the marriage of your son, the success of your son Peter, and the celebration of parents 9th wedding anniversary as advanced octogenarians.

It is a privilege to address the readers of your book, the have shared your experience of over close to 20 years and to congratulate you.

Sincerely,

Fred H. Hochberg, M.D.

DANA-FARBER/PARTNERS CANCERCARE

MASSACHUSETTS GENERAL HOSPITAL   DANA-FARBER CANCER INSTITUTE   BRIGHAM AND WOMEN'S HOSPITAL

4.

THE CONFERENCE

Now, what to do? Shortly thereafter, Mom, Aubrey and I made our first trip to Massachusetts General Hospital (the Mass General Zoo, more like it!).The wheelchair had to be brought from the hospital to the car. Aubrey lifted me into the wheelchair. Off we went to meet the world experts, Drs. Fred Hochberg and Amy Pruitt. Being wheeled through the halls (That place is huge!), I wondered how a human being could walk upright on two feet—the balance issue. People should be walking on all fours! Everyone hustling and bustling, walking fast. Doctors and nurses, students and volunteers, maintenance people and visitors. Everything was blurry. I felt like I was on a fast moving train, looking out the side window.

We met first with Dr. Pruitt. She had envelopes with X-rays all over the office, even on the floor. I was very impressed with her. I thought about how much she must know. And she was so young. Long hair tied back. I took a tape recorder and taped the meeting. Then we all met with Dr. Hochberg in a conference room and continued the taping (I first asked his permission).

Dr. Hochberg took over. Assuming the tumor was lymphoma, these were my options: One, just have radiation, and perhaps I would have less than one year of survival; two, go the experimental treatment route, receiving Methotrexate chemotherapy three times every three weeks, so that the chemo would go through the body, including the brain. It was necessary to receive an antidote, Calcium Leucovorin, at specifically scheduled times. This would remove Methotrexate from my body, but leave it in my brain. Then, I had to follow-up with radiation treatments. Dr. Hochberg said if we chose the experimental treatment, he did not know how long I would live, and that the longest living survivor of that treatment was four years at that time. After Mom asked Dr. Pruitt, if it were she, would she choose the latter? With her affirmative answer, we agreed. Wouldn't you?

My case is extremely rare. There are very few cases recorded in the annals of medical history; one doctor said 12, the other said 20. What makes it so rare is that if lymphoma is found in the brain, usually the primary site is in the bone marrow or elsewhere in the body. With me, it did start in the bone marrow, but my body was somehow able to take care of it from the neck down. I am told if one has to get brain cancer, this is a good one to get. (This must be the ultimate of looking at the bright side!) The entire meeting is on tape—all my mother's questions (she was always organized, and had everything written down) and all my outbursts of humor. I misplaced the tape for months, but when I found it and listened to it, it was like playing back a dream—or should I say a nightmare?!

I don't know how we sat there and discussed my fate. We (that is, my mom) made critical life choices.

Dr. Pruitt said, "Is there something in particular bothering you?" I said, "My image." "You mean your eyes, your vision?" I replied, "That too, but my image of myself."

The following conversation was taped during the conference at Mass General Hospital, September 1987. The conference began in Dr. Pruitt's office. Present were Dr. Pruitt, Mom, Aubrey and I. Then we four walked (I was pushed in a wheelchair, of course) to a different part of the hospital, where we met Dr. Hochberg in a special conference room. He proceeded to explain our options of treatment.

Conference Tape

Dr. Pruitt: OK. Let me just go over some of the things. A typical recommendation is to give the radiation to the back of the head, to a margin extending down into the neck a little bit, up to the rest of the head a bit, and that's been the conventional treatment. We're trying to get better results than that treatment alone affords. And, I'll state at the beginning, that no one knows for sure what the best drugs to do that are. The principals are that we can get more drugs into the right place, if it is given somewhat before the radiation.

Mom: What kind of…. How will this be administered?

Dr. Pruitt: One moment about that. Just a moment. There are two different drugs that have been studied. The better study of the two is something called Methotrexate. It's not a new drug; it's been around for years. Was actually developed as one of the first chemotherapy drugs for children with leukemia, and gets into the brain in a certain way by vein, into the rest of the body, in fairly high doses, so it gets into the brain in the kind of dose that we want. Then to protect the rest of the body 24 hours after that, an antidote to the drug is given, which essentially protects the body from ill effects of that medicine. You can do that very effectively. It's a several hour infusion of the drug, which in many places is done on an outpatient basis. We prefer to do it on an inpatient basis.

Mom: Will it be done here?

Dr. Pruitt: It would probably have to be done here. It could be done at Emerson.

Mom: How often would that be?

Dr. Pruitt: That would be once every three to four weeks.

Mom: M-m-m-m.

Dr. Pruitt: Probably for a few rounds. We will be looking at your Magnetic Resonance Imaging and/or your Cat Scan regularly during that interval, and to be followed by radiation therapy after three courses or so. If you would get into difficulty with new symptoms prior to that time, you would go on into the radiation…Now there is….

Mom: What are the side affects?

Dr. Pruitt: OK. The major side affect, as you can guess, is directed at cells that divide rapidly, and those cells, like blood cells, are affected by this medication. It turns out when the antidote is given, there is really little in the way of side affects on the rest of the body. And the major problem we are concerned with is a kidney problem. To that end, it's safer to be in the hospital to give you all kinds of things to make you drink a lot, and get flushed out quickly. This is only to….

Mom: Is this an overnight….

Dr. Pruitt: It's overnight.

Mom: …that you are talking about?

Dr. Pruitt: It might be actually a couple nights. We want to make sure the urine flow continues. And we give you the "rescue" (that's what it's called), the antidote at regular intervals for a few doses. We give you the rest in pills to take home. That's done two to three times, and done with the radiation, which you've already heard about, if given.

Mom: The radiation is an outpatient…?

Dr. Pruitt: That's right. That's right. And I guess I am not sure what facilities you will be recommended to..

Diane: Maybe it might be Waltham.

Dr. Pruitt: OK, where do you live?

Diane: Acton.

Dr. Pruitt: Well, this is a bit of a trek. It only takes two minutes a day. OK, the rationale behind this is to get as much drug throughout the area that might have cells, as possible, and to give the radiation to a localized area, where the bulk of the cells seem to be. I can't tell you that hundreds of people have had this treatment. I can tell you that 20 or so people have had this treatment at this hospital, and we are encouraged by very early results. There are not years worth of results to follow someone over time, but we know that the….tends to be better than radiation only. OK, what you would be getting into if you chose this route, would be only the commitment getting the medication the first couple of times…and you're still getting radiation anyway later.

Mom: How many treatments of radiation?

Dr. Pruitt: It would be likely on the order…probably 15 or as many as 20 separate treatments…It's daily for a couple minutes a day, almost always done….

Diane: It's the travel time.

Dr. Pruitt: That's right. It just takes a couple minutes…

Diane: They just zap you.

Dr. Pruitt: It just takes a couple minutes a day.

Diane: Should I be looking for a wig?

Dr. Pruitt: The area that will be treated will be primarily in the back, so there might be some initial hair loss, but it will come back. Uh-h-h, think the major issue involved around whether to elect to try an experimental treatment still, but which on the basis of preliminary information seems to be….

Diane: Working.

Dr. Pruitt: Working.

Mom: Preliminary. You mean 20 years?

Dr. Pruitt: Twenty people, not 20 years. Not just here, but in other hospitals. That's our experience here.

Mom: Is there any risk in this?

Dr. Pruitt: Well, I think there is. The immediate risk, as I mentioned to you, just the trauma of being in the hospital, and getting the things done.

Mom: Oh well.

Dr. Pruitt: We think we can give the medicine safely, and we're comfortable doing that.

Mom: Does that suppress the tumor, or does it…what does it do?

Dr. Pruitt: Well, we're going to wipe it out. That's the idea.

Mom: That's the idea.

Dr. Pruitt: That's the goal. It certainly…radiation will suppress it, too. But we have worries if only directed at this area, there could be microscopic cells in an area, that aren't in that area.

Mom: Is there a danger of radiation hurting the healthy cells?

Dr. Pruitt: Right. That's the major risk of radiation, period. With or without chemotherapy, the radiation has to be given in high doses to affect the bad cells, and is, therefore, in high enough doses, and it sometimes can affect the good cells, as well. Not immediately, but years down the road. It seems clear that radiation given first, and chemo second, that that intensifies the toxicity of the two, that they are worse. If we give it the other way, first chemotherapy, and then the radiation, then we are eliminating a lot of that additive.

Mom: Now, you call this chemotherapy, but they've been using chemotherapy…but they've been using a different drug.

Dr. Pruitt: They've been using chemotherapy for years for many different types of tumors.

Mom: M-m-hm.

Dr. Pruitt: Chemotherapy for brain tumors is relatively recent, and the reason is, it is tough to get medicine in the right place, in the right quantity. OK, chemotherapy with this drug is old, old, old, as old as chemotherapy is. It was essentially the first drug developed, and it turns out still to be one of the best. As I mentioned at the beginning, there are a couple other drugs being looked at…this one seems to be the best bet. What I would like to do, and I am going to give the people in the other building a call, have you come over there with me, meet the other people. Dr. Hochberg is the person who has primarily been doing this medication, and can give you some…I think he'll give you some…I don't happen to have any right now to read about it.

Diane: Read? (laughter)

Mom: All right now. After, say, she went through the drug treatment and radiation treatment, how do you know if she will need more treatments, or…?

Dr. Pruitt: Get regular scans.

Mom: Oh.

Dr. Pruitt: And various other tests on a routine basis.

Diane: (sarcastically) I just love taking tests.

Dr. Pruitt: Yeah, I'm sure. But, frankly, in this area, you are the best judge, meaning this is a sensitive area. You develop this numbness in your face or different…different movement of the right hand, you'd know something was up. It's not a very silent area of the head.

Diane: No.

Dr. Pruitt: If something happens in however some little way, you tend to know it.

Diane: You know about it.

Mom: Now, these treatments will affect her walking, make her walk better?

Dr. Pruitt: Well, we hope so. That's the idea.

Mom: That's the idea.

Dr. Pruitt: Oh, I see.

Mom: How about the eyes?

Dr. Pruitt: OK, the eyes. Clearly if the eyes aren't perfect, a little double vision is like a lot of double vision. You're still seeing two. You're either seeing one or you're not. I would imagine that of the various symptoms you have, the most difficult to clear up is probably the double vision. You might notice things getting closer together.

Diane: Uh-hmm. Uh-hmm.

Dr. Pruitt: Whether it would resolve entirely, I can't say.

Diane: The doctors want me to try without glasses, but I can't see…

Dr. Pruitt: I'm sure it's very…

Mom: Doesn't the…doesn't the eyes affect her balance?

Diane: Oh, yeah.

Dr. Pruitt: They both contribute, that's right.

Mom: She would have a problem, even if her right leg, you know, would be all right.

Dr. Pruitt: Yes.

Mom: She would still have a problem….

Dr. Pruitt: Yes.

Mom:…walking.

Dr. Pruitt: Though when you eliminate the double vision, it doesn't take away the balance issue altogether. So we know there is independently a problem with balance.

Mom: Oh, I see.

Aubrey: Could she get glasses…?

Dr. Pruitt: No, probably not. Certainly not at this point, 'cause we don't know how it's going to change.

Diane: Should I wait a few weeks?

Dr. Pruitt: Uh…months actually.

Diane: Months!

Dr. Pruitt: After all the things are over, if there is a fixed amount of double vision that isn't changing, then it makes sense to think about a prism in the glasses. Right now, if you got a prism, next week's prism would be different…

Mom: Yeah.

Dr. Pruitt: And it wouldn't be a good time…

Mom: It wouldn't be a good time.

Diane: See, the thing is, in the beginning I just had the blurred vision when I was diagnosed with labyrinthitis. And then worse towards the MRI test which diagnosed MS. In fact, just before the MRI. I started seeing double. Uh, now I look to the right, it just depends. If I look to the left, it's still blurry, because it just is. And I just see one. But when I look to the right, not only is it blurry, but it's double.

Dr. Pruitt: Yes. Right. Blurriness is probably an early stage of double vision,…

Diane: Uh-hmm.

Dr. Pruitt: and as it becomes more obvious to you that the images are separating, you no longer call it blurry; you call it double. Let me give the folks a call…

Diane: OK.

Dr. Pruitt:…before they disappear somewhere, and it would be certainly advantageous for you to talk to everybody.

Mom: Now are you talking to the technicians, or…?

Dr. Pruitt: It would be the doctors.

Diane: Dr. Hochberg.

Mom: Oh.

Dr. Pruitt: There is a radiation therapist, a surgeon, an oncologist,…(dials phone) This is Dr. Pruitt. May I speak with Dr. Hochberg, please?…

Mom: All right now. Is she supposed to be taking vitamins?

Dr. Pruitt: I have no objection.

Mom: No objection.

Dr. Pruitt: In fact, the antidote to this other medicine, should be designed together as a form of a vitamin, so you'll only be getting it two times.

Diane: I have some from a….

Aubrey: Why would she not?

Diane: …nutritionist. Dr. Vaillant told me.

Aubrey: Why would she not?

Dr. Pruitt: (on phone) Hello. I'm sitting with a woman I spoke to you about earlier. Do you have a moment to go? I have all her films and things, and I think it would be useful…OK. OK, yeah, thanks. (hangs up phone) OK, why would she not? Well, that's a very good question. You would not because no one can stand up to her and prove to her that it's a better course.

Diane: I have already started taking some from this nutritionist, this marine oil and riboflavin…

Mom: She can take it with any medication?

Diane:….antioxidant.

Dr. Pruitt: OK, those are all good theories. Again, I'm not standing up by saying I've proved my theories either…

Diane: But, it's not going to hurt me if I take it.

Dr. Pruitt: No. No. It's not going to hurt you. And it can never hurt that you were in good shape to start out with. Should we choose not to do it, because she chose not to do something experimental…OK, now all of us here are of a mind, when we look at this data years down the road, we're going to say, "Uh-ha, this was the right thing to do, but I can't prove that in 1987". She can say, "Nobody puts me in the hospital, and puts me on intravenous lines, and takes up any more of my time than he has to, unless he can prove it. That's why she would choose not to. OK, I think the toxicity is clearly acceptable.

Mom: Now, if you had it, you would do it?

Dr. Pruitt: Yeah, I would.

Mom: You would.

Dr. Pruitt: Would. And I think that...then again, that's also a matter of a lot of me. Many people will tell me "I will do anything, though, if it's never been done before, or it's only been...." And that's fine, and others will say, "If you can tell me two years from now, then that is a better route to go." Uh, the problem with that approach, of course, that it seems safer to give the drug first, and not years from now.

Aubrey: So, basically, that's your...this is your recommendation.

Dr. Pruitt: My recommendation is that you're a young person, who despite the location of this thing, has come through the surgery very well, and you're still improving, and we go for what is not crazy, but sane, and the most aggressive approach. I think, but that's not telling you that you really shouldn't. I think the more correct thing for you to do is to do everything as soon as possible. OK.

Mom: OK, now what if she improves and everything goes smoothly, when will this begin?

Dr. Pruitt: Probably...next week.

Mom: Probably this...

Dr. Pruitt: I would have...we'll speak to the crew downstairs. We have to get the logistics, as such. We have to get a specific bed and a specific place where the nurses know how to do this, too, and then it's just a question of timing.

Mom: All right now. Will she have any resistance to colds or flu or anything like this?

Dr. Pruitt: We hope there won't be anything from this medicine, because we are going to give an antidote to it. You're on steroids, which lowers your resistance to things. One of the ideas, that's what this does, is to get you off the steroids, or at least lower the dose as rapidly as possible.

Aubrey: The steroids do lower her resistance...?

Dr. Pruitt: They do. They do.

Aubrey: ...like to a common cold, or...

Dr. Pruitt: In theory, yes. In practice I'll have to say you can measure colds per winter, or something like that, but over the....it's really more of a duration thing. It's not how much you're taking today, but how much you have to take over a period of months that really…

Mom: She's always warm, you know. I'll be cold, and she feels like she's warm. Is there anything…

Diane: No, no, Mom. In the hospital, it's cold.

Mom: Maybe she's a little worried, you know.

Dr. Pruitt: I think the thyroid functions in there are OK. That's the only major explanation for that. Let's uh…in fact, we're about as far from that place as we can be, while being in the same institution. So, let's go out on our trek, and meet everybody over there, and think about it some more….Hopefully, it will be more or less the same thing.

Mom: You know my son was really worried about the consultation today.

Dr. Pruitt: OK, that's fair, but we do send him a note anyhow.

Mom: Well, thank you.

In Conference Room

Dr. Hochberg: We're going to make certain assumptions. The first assumption is that Dr. Moore has found, and that the neuro-pathologist…will confer that this is a….lymphoma, which is a tumor that starts in the body, shows itself in the brain, and therefore has to be treated in the brain tissue. Now, I tell you in that way, because it is an unusual tumor, and really starts in the bone marrow, and yet, in certain people, we've seen about a hundred and twenty now. Even though it starts in the bone marrow, the body seems to take care of it from the neck down, but doesn't take care of it in the brain tissue. Now we know certain things about it. We know most people do very well receiving steroids, Decadron, or…

Dr. Pruitt: Got better on its own once.

Mom: That's what she didn't understand.

Diane: I was diagnosed with labyrinthitis.

Dr. Hochberg: Well, that happens. And the reason…I'll tell you the reason it happens in a second. But, to clear up one thing first. No one comes into the hospital and has this diagnosis made easily. So, if you wonder why labyrinthitis, why Multiple Sclerosis, why they said it was a viral infection. It's always complicated. So, they, your physicians, did as much as they could….

Diane: We understand that.

Dr. Hochberg: Even if you would have come here on Day One, it would have been the same.

Diane: Uh-mmm.

Dr. Hochberg: Now the reason that it possibly went away. We think there are two stages of this. One which is a single growth of many types of cells, and the cells might be viewed as having, one cell has a red hat, one cell has a blue hat, one cell has a green hat. And, over the course of time, these cells only select the cells with red hats, which are the ones that stay around. So the reason we think why steroids make it better, and sometimes it goes away, is because it starts out as many types of cells, and becomes one type of cell.

Diane: (I had no idea what he was talking about with the hats!) I was never under any medication at first, only Meclizine and…

Dr.Hochberg: I've heard those stories where people literally, without any reason…One lady, five years after her initial experience, had it come back, even though it had gone away by itself, so sometimes it will. Now, that's the relatively good news. The bad news is the fact that we know an awful lot about this tumor, and some of the information we have is not very exciting. Number one. Even though the steroids have worked. they're not going to work forever, so that we can't assume that by giving you steroids is going to cure this. So, we have to take the steroids, and push them to the side.

Diane: The Decadron.

Dr. Hochberg: The Decadron.

Diane: When would that….

Dr.Hochberg: It's not so much a matter of when, but simply to adjust your thinking to the fact that steroids are not going to be the final answer for you.

Diane: Well, we know that.

Dr. Hochberg: OK, secondly we believe that radiation therapy, although it's very good, is not the final answer either. And the reason is that when I look over the information from the United States, where they gave radiation treatment to 45 people through last month, the best that they could hope for was one year's survival, given radiation treatment alone. So, radiation is probably good, but in and of itself, given alone, it's not going to solve the situation.

Diane: By itself.

Dr. Hochberg: By itself. So, we're going to use radiation, but we're going to make it part of a combined approach to this. Now, the reason you don't have to remember this, is that I wrote an eight or nine page explanation, which goes over everything we're going to talk about today. And I'd like you to read it, even before we make any decisions. I want you to read it and go through questions with Dr. Pruitt, so that you feel comfortable about everything. And only then can we make some plans....Now, let me show you three things, if I can, on the blackboard. We have this all spelled out. The first is that we know this started somewhere in your body, and we have to then treat the rest of the body in some fashion. Otherwise, we have the danger of having it reseed from the body to the brain. So, we have to treat this. The second is that even though we know it's in the back of the brain now, we run the danger of having this spread elsewhere in the brain, so we just can't treat the place we see it. We have to treat the entire brain tissue.

Diane: Uh-hmm.

Dr. Hochberg: OK, and the third is, we have to make sure that the fluid that covers the brain is also treated, because sometimes it becomes involved with these cells. Well, OK?

Diane: U-hmm.

Dr. Hochbertg: Now, as a result, what we've begun to do is give a medication, which is called Methotrexate. And what we do...this is all written down for you, so you don't have to worry about it. My secretary is going to bring over a copy of the written material. We would have you come into the hospital for about two and a half days. We'd give you a large amount of fluid by mouth. We'd give you the Methotrexate four hours by vein.

Diane: It's very difficult for me to take fluid by mouth.

Dr. Pruitt: You need to not be dehydrated.

Diane: OK.

Dr. Hochberg: All right. We give you the Methotrexate by vein. Then we do something very clever. We reverse the Methotrexate. The Methotrexate will enter the body, enter the brain, enter the spinal fluid.

Diane: How will I feel when I'm lying there when all this is happening? Will I feel like...

Dr. Pruitt: Different people feel different ways.

Dr. Hochberg: The worst you're going to feel is washed out.

Diane: Oh, well. That's nothing.

Dr. Hochberg: Nausea and vomiting, we do not see it.

Diane: That's good. I can give you a good dose of that! (laughter)

Dr. Hochberg: Really. You'll read about everything in this paper. Everyone's hair doesn't fall out; maybe your hair will. People don't have nausea and vomiting, but maybe you will. But, in general, the worst I have seen, with the exception of one lady who was seventy-five years of age, who became confused that night because of the fluid…The worst I've seen is that people feel like a dishrag.

Diane: I can handle dishrag.

Dr. Hochberg: OK. Anyway, we give this material. It goes through these systems, and then we give the antidote to reverse the material.

Diane: Uh-hmm.

Dr. Hochberg: Now, we probably will give this every three weeks, but I'm not sure yet. Because one of the things we're beginning to find is that we can get away with giving it every week. And because of that, we may make it easier on you. There's no reason to space this apart. We do know we're only going to give you three treatments. The likelihood is that nine out of 10 patients will have their disease disappear…But, even if it disappears, we're then going to go ahead and give you radiation.

Diane: Uh-hmm.

Dr. Hochberg: We'll combine this with radiation to try to stamp this out. Now, the thing you want to know is, is this thing going to be cured forever, or are you going to be 80 years old when I see you next time? And I can't tell you that, because the longest we followed anybody is four years. One young lady. But, it's not a common tumor, so I can't tell you we've treated 150 patients. We have only treated about 12.

Dr. Pruitt: Altogether, I think that it's a total of about 20 people or so…

Mom: Yes. Yes.

Dr. Hochberg: Now, you might say, "What else is there in the United States?" Well, if you start calling around, you're going to get our name again. So, there are other approaches that are available, but in my mind, there is none that is so clearly better that makes any sense to move on elsewhere.

Diane: That's good news.

Dr. Hochberg: So, what I am going to do is give you this paper to read. Make a couple copies of it, show it to local doctors, sit down and discuss with Dr. Pruitt, so that...

Dr. Pruitt:....You know more or less what we're talking about.

Mom: Mm-hmm.

Dr. Hochberg: Make sure you're comfortable with it all, then I'm happy to sit down and discuss with you if you have any questions. "What floor will I be on? What time of day will I have to come into the hospital? Can I have a private room? Who's my nurse going to be?"

Mom: Oh, those are...

Dr. Hochberg: "Which arm are they going to put my intravenous in?"

Mom:....those are minor things. (laughter) Those are minor.

Dr. Hochberg: I want people to feel comfortable with this, because it's very complicated, and if you say...if you, if you know, if you go to your local doctor, and you say to him, they're probably going to do this. I would think the word you would have to use is "experimental."

Mom: All right. What I want to ask is...now...if she agrees to this...which I think she will...uh...Dr. Pruitt thought it might be in a week or two, but what if you don't get your slides back, and get the complete...?

Dr. Pruitt: Well, I'm going to start calling, but they should be ready, actually. Some of the slides take a little bit longer. What we usually know...

Mom: It will be two weeks tomorrow since she had surgery.

Dr. Pruitt: What we need to know is that the category of the disease we're talking about is lymphoma, and not some other type of cell...OK. All of what we said doesn't matter, if this isn't lymphoma. I'm assuming that Dr. Hochberg has told you, also, that it's lymphoma. What type of lymphoma is of more relevance to us...

Mom: Uh-hmm. Uh-hmm.

Dr. Pruitt:...than to you in making the decision.

Dr. Hochberg: Well, since you asked the question, I think that what we're going to do...

Dr. Pruitt: I'm going to call them...

Dr. Hochberg: Better than that we are going to send you out there.

Diane: Send us where?

Dr. Hochberg: Right to the person who has this, and you're going to literally ask his secretary for the slides and report. Dr. Pruitt will write down

where it is, because, otherwise, we run the risk of being five days before
we receive it.

Mom: (to Diane) Uh-h, are you able to sit up?

Diane: I'm fine.

Mom: You're fine?

Dr. Pruitt: Let me call their office today, and make sure they're done.

Mom: Where is the pathology?...

Dr. Hochberg: UMASS

Diane: I'm fine.

Dr. Hochberg: You don't have to go. (laughter in room)

Mom: I'm not from here. I don't even know...

Dr. Hochberg: Well, you go...

Mom: I'm from California.

Diane: (in Mae West voice) Just put me in the car, and treat me like a queen!

Dr. Hochberg: One of you goes, and let Dr. Pruitt make the phone call;
they'll listen to you. We have a nice relationship.

Mom: Is it...is it in this area?

Diane: No.

Mom: Oh, it's in...

Dr. Hochberg: It's about an hour's drive. (Everyone looks at Aubrey.)
(laughter)

Aubrey: Sure, hey, if they'll give it to me.

Diane...go home and take a nap.

Dr. Pruitt: Be sure, in fact, that they're all there before you...and it doesn't
have to be yesterday, so...

Dr. Hochberg: So, my secretary will bring this over to you for you all to read.
I'd like you to call into Dr. Pruitt or my office. I'll give you a card. Call us
toward the middle of the week, say Thursday or so. Think about it, and
what we'll try to do, if we have the slides, is to begin this next week.

Diane: Sounds good to me.

Mom: Now all right. We come to where?

Dr. Pruitt: OK.

Dr. Hochberg: They'll get ready for you.

Mom: Oh, all right.

Dr. Pruitt: Where and when you come...the logistics of the bed, and all that
sort of thing...as soon as we have the slides, we can...

Mom: (to Aubrey) Do you know where he's talking about?

Aubrey: UMASS?
Mom: Yeah, because I don't know anything from nothing here.
Aubrey: Oh, yeah, we'll shoot up and get it.
Diane: UMASS. Amherst? Amherst?
Dr. Pruitt: No.
Dr. Hochberg: Worcester. I don't have a phone number.
Dr. Pruitt: Not quite that bad…
Dr. Hochberg: It's quite near us.
Mom: Well, he can give you an address and everything.
Diane: You know what I'm gonna do, Mom. I'm gonna stop this. (referring to the tape)
Mom: Well, you're getting all the paper anyway.

============================

Following is the consent form, containing all the information which Dr. Hochberg spoke about it in the conference, which I had to sign prior to treatment. I signed it because Mom thought this was the best thing for me to do, and also because neither could I read it, nor listen to it with any comprehension.

Massachusetts General Hospital
Medical Research Form

Title of Project: Treatment of Primary Lymphoma of the Nervous System with High Dose Methotrexate Prior to Irradiation
Principal Investigator: Dr. Fred Hochberg

PURPOSE OF RESEARCH

Background: I have been told by my doctor that I am suffering from a brain tumor, which is called a primary lymphoma of the nervous system. Previous attempts to treat this tumor have included the use of surgery, and radiation therapy, as well as chemotherapy. The surgery and radiation experiences have not been successful in curing this disease. The use of a drug called Methotrexate has brought about responses in some patients. However, no cures have been seen with this drug when given alone. This drug has also been used to treat lymphoma when it involves other areas of the body. However, when this drug is used to treat lymphoma of the brain, it requires a greater amount of Methotrexate, than what is ordinarily used for lymphoma localized in other parts of the body. Since there is such a large amount of drug used, an antidote called Leucovorin will be used to remove the Methotrexate from the blood stream, while allowing enough of the drug to remain in the brain where it is needed. The drug has been used for many years. Neither the drug nor the technique of administration is new. What is new is the drug to treat this tumor, and then to give radiation therapy after completion of three cycles of Methotrexate. The doctors propose to give me this Methotrexate by vein every three weeks for three times before I have radiation therapy, which will be started three weeks after the third and final dosage of Methotrexate. By receiving the medication by vein, the doctors hope to provide enough drug to kill off the tumor in my brain and any sites in which it may be hiding. By giving it every three weeks for three times, this will hopefully cause most of the tumor cells to die. The remainder can be treated with radiation therapy. This approach involves clinical research—an effort to find a more successful way to possibly cure this tumor. We hope to improve this situation with the addition of the Methotrexate to radiation.

PROCEDURES

The doctors expect to administer the drug every three weeks. Three separate courses of drug will be given in this way over a 9-week period. Three weeks after the last course, radiation therapy will begin. The administration of the drug will continue for three treatments and radiation therapy will be given, even if there is no longer clear evidence of the tumor by CAT Scan, as well as not further neurological symptoms present.

Each time I am evaluated, a CAT Scan, a brain wave test and eye examination, in addition to the usual neurological examination will be performed. The doctors will discuss performing a lumbar puncture for cerebral spinal fluid examination for tumor cells before each chemotherapy. In addition, initial laboratory data will be collected to aid in modification of the amount of drug to be administered. There may be pain and a black and blue mark at the site of the veinpuncture for the blood tests. The drug will be given by vein over a four-hour period of time. As soon as the medication is run in, the doctors will allow it to distribute throughout my body. Four hours later, the doctors will start an antidote for the medication to remove it from the place where the drug is no longer needed. This will be done by using a drug called Leucovorin which is a potent agent for neutralizing the possible immediate toxic effects that the Methotrexate may have on the tissue that helps produce blood in my bone marrow. It will be done by administering the Leucovorin for 8 doses, by vein, 6 hours apart. This will then be followed by an additional 4 doses by mouth. Presumably, although it may be removed from my blood stream in this fashion, certain amounts of Methotrexate will stay in my brain and spinal fluid where the lymphoma may still be hiding. If this approach is successful, the doctors will repeat it two more times, three weeks apart. The doctors also may choose to give me corticosteroids on an as needed basis, medication which is meant to help in controlling the swelling in the brain.

I will be required to be hospitalized for the Methotrexate administration for approximately two days.

The National Cancer Institute will pay for the cost of the Methotrexate, and I or my insurance will be required to cover any other expenses incurred in the hospital or for office visits.

It will be necessary to follow me for several years, and to obtain a neurologic exam and CAT Scan every 4 months to determine that the tumor remains in remission. After radiation, a lumbar puncture for cerebral spinal fluid will be performed every four months for one year in search for any remaining tumor cells.

RISKS AND DISCOMFORTS

The administration of this drug will not cause me pain; however, it can cause nausea and vomiting. It also may result in a decrease of white blood cells which can lead to infection and/or bleeding.

Although the drug has been used safely under many circumstances, it carries the possibility of some side effects, such as diarrhea or inflammatory lesions in my mouth called stomatitis. Clearly, there may be difficulty with the intravenous infusion. I may be one of the rare patients who is allergic to the drug. If I am allergic to Methotrexate, my liver may suffer damage or seizures may occur.

Should the drug cause a lowering of my blood cell count, or cause damage to my kidneys, these may cause doctors to halt administration of the drug or alter the dose. Rarely the drug, in combination with radiation therapy has produced damage to the white matter of the brain (which results in seizures).

However, the radiation cannot be given during the administration of the Methotrexate, but rather three weeks after the infusion, in hopes of reducing this risk even more. The doctors will obtain CAT Scans and brain wave tests, so that the doctors may anticipate this damage before it occurs. I UNDERSTAND THAT IT IS ABSOLUTELY NECESSARY THAT THE ANTIDOTE (LEUCOVORIN) MUST BE ADMINISTERED EXACTLY AS PLANNED TO AVOID POTENTIALLY FATAL SIDE EFFECTS TO MY BLOOD FORMING SYSTEM.

This drug will almost certainly cause damage to a developing fetus. If there is any possibility of pregnancy, I will be excluded from this protocol. If there is any possibility of pregnancy, a pregnancy test must be performed, and I should consult my doctor about pregnancy prevention during this therapy. If I have been involved in any research studies or, medical diagnostic or therapeutic activity in the recent past, I should inform my doctor.

BENEFITS

It is not known if the size of the tumor will decrease as a result of my participation in this therapy, although it is hoped that this will occur. The therapy brings together two logical approaches to the treatment of this tumor—drug therapy, followed by irradiation. Others may benefit if this approach is found to be very effective.

ALTERNATIVES TO PARTICIPATION

There are alternatives to receiving Methotrexate before radiation. My tumor may be treated with steroids, radiation therapy and Methotrexate after radiation alone, or I may choose to be treated with steroids and radiation alone.

5.

DISABLED AND DEPENDENT

Home services were set up for me: a physical therapist, Kathy; an occupational therapist, Sue; and a visiting nurse, Pam. Soon I was getting my own breakfast ready at night for the next morning. It took too much energy for me to both set up for breakfast, and eat it, also. At the suggestion of Sue, we purchased a red multi-shelved basket on wheels to transport things from one place to another around the kitchen. Pushing the cart around, and handling a walker at the same time was almost impossible!

I had to have a shower bar installed in my bathroom upstairs, and also a shower chair. I couldn't take a shower by myself. I also had to have another bar installed next to the toilet in the downstairs bathroom, and have railings put outside for the steps leading from the garage into the family room. Not only did I have to deal with adjusting to, and using these helpful devices, but I had to come to grips that I was *disabled, handicapped*! It's the image. I never pictured myself this way—so dependent.

Karl and John, friends from where I used to work, were always here, putting in bars, or fixing plumbing or something. Also, other people at work contributed their time and efforts into various projects. One day Karl and John brought in a freezer, from an anonymous donor. Mom couldn't stay forever, so she would cook every day and fill it up.

I don't know how she managed to do everything: the hospital, the doctors and nurses, the kids, Boswell, the dog, (She brushed him a million times a day.), the shopping, the cooking, the laundry, and ME! (That's a lot in itself!) She had to greet the neighbors, and also turn them away when it got to be too much.

I would have to take naps several times a day. I also got into a ritual where I had to sleep 3:30 p.m. to 6:30 p.m. upstairs without phone or visitors or any noise. I would then get up for dinner and go back to sleep again at 7:30 p.m. Sometimes I felt so wiped out, that I couldn't wait for 7:15 p.m. to get here, but I tried to be strong, and stay up. It took me about 20 minutes to get ready for bed.

It felt forever, taking each step with my walker. Walker, left foot, right foot. Walker, left foot, right foot. My best foot forward. That's how they taught me in the hospital. I would have given *anything* to walk through my kitchen, unassisted and without holding onto any counters or walls.

It was hard for me to do the simplest things. To brush my teeth and wash up, I had to lean my walker and my hips against the sink. I had to clutch my legs to the toilet seat to keep from falling. Any bathroom duties were difficult, even taking the paper off the roll. Having my period was an extra effort. Also, it was hard to get dressed. Months later, when I was able to put on my pierced earrings, that was a "biggie!"

6.

CHEMOTHERAPY

Back to Mass General in three weeks for chemotherapy. In the meantime, I had to keep taking Decadron (sounds like "decadent" to me), liquid potassium, and a few other beauties. My mother had to administer these drugs to me, because I was unable to unscrew the cap, or would have had a hard time counting out the pills.

There is too much to say about Mass General to say it all here. It's a real ZOO, as I mentioned. A lot of waiting for your room. One time I had to wait so long, my mother strongly insisted they get me a bed. They did. In the orthopedic ward. I was sort of misplaced, and at first, they couldn't find me!

Aubrey always took Mom and me. Same old routine. Drop off. Get the wheelchair. Park the car. Go to the desk. Show your card. Be admitted. Meet your nurse (I had so many, I can't count.) I definitely had my favorites. Some were better able to handle the stresses brought on by the nursing shortage. Therefore, sometimes there was a lot of waiting for my bedpan.

So, what is chemotherapy? I can tell you what it was for me. It meant spending two-and-a-half or three days in the hospital (depending on the expediency in finding a wheelchair at the time I was ready to go home). Soon we learned to confiscate one right before I was discharged. Chemotherapy also meant packing a hospital bag with all my personal things. I always needed my granola and a couple bananas. A big teddy bear, my friend, Judy, bought me, became my constant companion. It would ride with me in the wheelchair, and its neck would always get stuck in the bed railing.

Chemotherapy was four hours of a liquid, which looked like dark urine dripping into my vein. It meant drinking a glass of water every hour. I have always had a hard time drinking a lot of liquid, so this was a real challenge! I had to keep track of how much I drank, so I ticked off marks on a paper towel with a pencil. Not to be outdone, sometimes I would stay ahead of the game and drink two glasses in one hour. The granola helped make me thirsty. I ate day and night. I was awake most of the night, and so I was eating, too. Soon, with the medication and eating, I was 20 pounds heavier, and I was even feeling worse about myself. The best part is I never felt nauseous, or lost my hair. I did have some mouth sores, but not bad. I took something called "Swish and Spit," and that's exactly what I did.

Calcium Leucovorin. I had to take this at regular times by mouth, even when I got home. Mom and I both set alarms for 3 a.m., as it was imperative, to prevent possible fatal complications, I took this medication on time to clear the body of the Methotrexate, while leaving it in the brain. I can't get over the strength and stamina of my mother—no way could I have made it without her loving care. After three more weeks I would go again to have chemo. Same routine, but always something different happening.

I was missing my kids. First of all, when I got home, I didn't have the strength or energy to be the mother I wanted to be. Secondly, I had to go to bed so early, so I would miss all the comings and goings and late night talk. Now, August, I usually nap in the afternoon, and I stay up until 1 a.m. Peter's curfew is at midnight, so this gives me a chance to be with him, if the only thing we do is watch TV together. Besides, I've always liked the night life. I do some of my best work at night. I think better. Sometimes, I seem to walk better.

One thing for sure—I knew I always had to go back to Baker 5, the cancer ward at Mass General. My third time, my last trip to Baker 5, when I was discharged I felt as if I was getting out of prison. Taking that next step. One step closer to control and independence.

7.

DIANE'S BUDDY SYSTEM

After that, November 5, my mom went back to California. I was scared, because I still felt helpless, like a baby. I knew she had to leave sometime, but how would I manage? Before she left, we approached one of my friends to organize help for me—someone who was smart, dependable, organized and caring. This would be Joyce Johnson. She, with the help of Ellen Valade, organized "Diane's Buddy System."

This would be the support group that would beat all support groups anywhere, any time. About 75 people comprised of neighbors, friends, church, Emerson Hospital Auxiliary, and my cleaning lady took care of me. It was mostly organized with a captain and five crew people for each day. Each person had shifts and would report to the captain. The Auxiliary women would cook for me on some days, and Joyce, Ellen, and my friend, Valerie, would arrange with others to have meals on all the remaining days. I had a large write-on-wipe-off calendar on the wall in my kitchen, so Joyce kept the food schedule up to date. This lasted nine months. I am not just talking about a main meal; I'm talking, in addition, bread, croissants, salad, salad dressing, dessert, flowers, and hugs.

People were scheduled to take me for radiation. I never had to worry about anything. People gave my kids rides to their activities, got groceries, did laundry, and took trash out. Some felt comfortable buzzing about the house, taking care of details. Others were helpful in keeping me company and listening.

My cleaning lady, who referred to herself as George, did everything from doing my laundry to cleaning out the dog's eating area. I didn't have to tell her what to do, and I was not able to anyway. She was just very aware. I am so lucky to have had (and I still do) the support and outpouring of love from everyone. I was meeting neighbors I hadn't even met before. Everyone was talking to each other, and they were truly focused on helping me, while at the same time, unknowingly, bonding with each other. Unbelievable teamwork!

What to do with my time soon became an issue. People brought me large print books, but my eyes were not even good enough for that. I also did not have the energy or coordination to turn the pages. It wasn't worth the effort. A great idea—talking books from the library, but this was too passive for me to take for long. Couldn't get into the soaps. Never did before. An Amos & Andy tape won over any inspirational tape. I guess I needed comedy so that I could laugh.

People were praying for me all over the world: California, Massachusetts, Florida, Ohio, Nebraska, and in-between. In Sweden and Germany. There were prayers said on Sunday in many churches. A third-grade class, taught by my friend, Judy York, in Maynard, Massachusetts, prayed for me every single day. Sometimes, when the teacher would forget, they would remind her. Each of the kids made cards for me. Love and support and prayers. People coming together. That is one of the main reasons I am where I am today. And I will be forever grateful.

8.

RADIATION

What is radiation? On November 24, I had my first treatment at Waltham Hospital. Previously, I had met at Mass General with Dr. Lingood, and then had to meet with the technician to measure my head, etc., to determine exactly what part of my head needed to be zapped, and what part needed to be protected with lead blocks. The technician had to shave my head, slightly over each ear, and mark it permanently with a pen, so that I could be quickly lined up when I went in for radiation.

Entering the waiting room felt a little eerie, for I had just been here a few months ago with my friend, Jane, who had just recently died of cancer. Same nurse. Same everything. It was very scary!

It was my turn. I was wheeled into the room. Helped onto the table. Big ominous-looking machine. The technician located the two dots on my head, put in the plate with the lead block on it, and taped my head down with masking tape from one end of the table to the other. On her way out, she would say, "OK now, hold still." Then the heavy door would close with a loud bang. The buzzing noise would begin. After a few appointments of radiation, I started counting. It took about 20 seconds for each side of my head (she would have to put another block in when she switched sides.) On second six, there was a bright flashing light, and then about 14 more seconds. This would happen for 17 visits.

What amazed me was the manner in which patients went in and came out. It was a job. I'm not saying it was "cold," but different people were having different parts of their bodies zapped, and you might as well be having an appointment at the dentist's office. Of course, this was much more serious, but yet it was just people doing their jobs. Doing it, day in and day out.

I saw the nutritionist and the doctor once a week. I guess I was eating right because I gained over 20 pounds! I was not too happy about this, but I was told that this was not the time to go on a diet, and I definitely did not want to be a skinny cancer patient. When I started to cry, the doctor asked me why I was crying. With my crying voice, I yelled out, "Because I'm fat!" I think the doctor thought I was crazy because I was more upset with my weight gain and image of myself than I was about the tumor. He rolled his eyes and glanced up at the nurse, with a look as if to say, "What am I going to do with her?"

Previously, Dr. Lingood, the radiation doctor at Mass General, said I would probably start losing my hair during the third week of radiation. Gosh, right on time! I was told by the nurse that I would probably continue to lose it for one or two weeks after radiation. But, nobody said anything about two months!

I asked, "So where does the hair go? Is it like a dog shedding? Does it all end up on your pillow one morning?" Everywhere, sort of. A little bit every day on your pillow, in your bed, in the shower, in the sink, on your clothes, just plain everywhere. It started coming out in clumps. O-o-oh scary!! Pretty soon the *process* of losing my hair became more devastating and stressful than the actual *loss* of it.

I was so tempted to have my head shaved, and dispense with this gradual torture, but I didn't have the guts. Plus, I kept thinking, "This is going to be it; they said one or two weeks." But, the hair just kept falling out, until I was almost totally bald, save a few strands of hair. Dr. Lingood said that I would at least lose 90 percent, but my hair was so thick, I thought it wouldn't happen to me.

I wondered how it would feel to wash a bald head—it's just like washing the head of a baby. Except it feels weird if it's your own, and you're used to having enough hair for three people. Are you supposed to brush your hair? I mean scalp?

The radiation hurt my scalp. I had to use a medicated cream on my head. It felt as if I had a burn. And something strange was happening—my face was actually getting tanned. In fact, someone asked me if I had been on vacation!

At the end of my treatment, I had progressed to using a cane. The cane became a part of me, and I took it almost everywhere I went. Only one time do I remember leaving it home, and after this experience, I never forgot it again!

My friend, Valerie, was taking me for a ride. She decided to get the car washed. The car derailed and was stuck in the middle of the car wash. The water was still spraying, and the brushes were still brushing. I'm not fond of car washes anyway, but under normal circumstances, I knew I would soon get through. But, here we were stuck, and here I was without my cane. No control. No independence. I told myself to be patient, and this would not last forever. I visualized someone carrying me out of the car. I really have a hard time being so dependent. I felt scared and helpless. (Note: In retrospect, I probably would have been scared, even if I were as healthy as could be.)

9.

STARTING OVER

"It is no disgrace starting over. It is usually an opportunity, for some men never get that second chance." Anonymous

It's hard for me to start anything over. (I used to hate reviewing in school; it was so boring.) One day when my mother was with me, we were both sitting at the kitchen table. She was cutting up vegetables, and I was trying to write my ABC's in a Snoopy penmanship tablet. I became frustrated and started to cry. She said, "Why are you crying?" I said, "I'm almost 44 years old, and I can't even write my ABC's. I had lost a lot of coordination in my right hand, with also the right side of my body being the affected side. I felt this happening, even before surgery.

My birthday is November 21. A lot of friends and neighbors brought presents and good wishes. One neighbor, Lynn, put a large birthday card on the door for people to sign, and also a sign that said, "Tease me about my age and I'll beat you with my cane."

Also, Dr. Vaillant (Dr. V.), my primary care doctor, happened to be here on this day. He came to the house regularly, from the very beginning. He didn't examine me as a doctor would in his office: blood pressure, etc., but he sat for about an hour and talked to me. I observed him observing me. He gave me so much encouragement and support. He always told me how well I was doing. I needed so much to see him, and I always looked forward to his visits. He always gave me a big hug before he left.

Following is an account of my daily journal suggested by him. He told me to keep a journal, mainly to improve my fine motor coordination. Much later, when I attended a seminar by Dr. Bernie Siegel, author of "Love, Medicine and Miracles" and, "Peace, Love, and Healing," I had the opportunity to meet him and give him this manuscript. I have a photo of him giving me a hug, and I noticed his large belt buckle that said "BERNIE." He wrote me a note at the bottom of my letter to him in large letters with a purple marker, saying, "Your doctor helped save your life by telling you to keep a journal." I framed the original letter which I have displayed in my house, and framed a copy for Dr.V., which I think is hanging in his office. (Flipping through the pages of my actual journal, one can see the progression and striking improvement in my handwriting.)

Monday, November 23, 1987

Today I'm starting to write again. What a pain in the neck! Dr. V. wants me to write a little bit every day.

Tuesday, November 24

I just finished my breakfast. Today is my first day of radiation. I'm scared, even though I know I have gone through the worst part.

Wednesday, November 25

Treatment #2. I'm more tired than usual; I can expect that from the treatments. Oh well, only two-and-a-half weeks to go. No nausea, just very tired.

Thursday, November 26

Happy Thanksgiving! Today will be a better day than yesterday, which was a real downer. The kids are going to The Rusty Scupper Restaurant with their father, and I will be having dinner with Aubrey (meal cooked by a friend from the hospital auxiliary). I love it when I have a day off from my treatments. 2:25pm: Aubrey and I are just finishing a little lunch. Today Acton won their football game against Maynard. The kids went and got soaked from the rain.

Friday, November 27

It would help if I could see. Today is Treatment #3. Aubrey is taking me today. I'm told I shouldn't expect any improvement for a few weeks. The treatments really tire me out.

Saturday, November 28

Another day, another dollar. No treatment today—yeah! Judy was here for breakfast. She might take the kids shopping in Framingham today. David wants to look at pool tables.

Sunday, November 29

Today is a gray day outside. It's supposed to rain. Nothing really planned for the day. Going to take it easy. All next week I have treatments. Trying to take things in stride.

Monday, November 30

Let's see. Today Peter and David have basketball tryouts. Treatment #4. I put a bra on for the first time in months. It's 9:30 a.m. I'm going to take a little rest. If I position my head and eyes a certain way, I see single, not double.

Tuesday, December 1

Treatment #5. Valerie takes me today. Yesterday Joyce and I stopped in the Waltham Hospital gift shop to look at some terrycloth turbans—yucko! Ugly pastel color of blue, pink and yellow—maybe for summer, but not now. I may not need any turbans anyway!

Wednesday, December 2

Ellen is here folding clothes right now. She found my pink socks I've been "looking" for. Treatment #6. I swear they fry my brain. I can smell it. Yesterday I started writing my checks.

Thursday, December 3

Treatment #7. Yesterday I walked from the car to the hospital lobby (with my walker). Tonight Peter goes to the RUSH rock concert. And basketball continues. I want to go to the kids' games.

Friday, December 4

Treatment #8. Yesterday I didn't use the walker. Today it is snowing. I think I will use my walker so my driver does not have a heart attack. Today I did twenty minutes on the rowing machine. Dr. V. was here yesterday. He said I'm doing great. I guess I needed that.

Saturday, December 5

How the time flies when you're having fun! A day off from treatment. Peter made the varsity basketball team, and had an eight o'clock practice. David will find out on Monday. No problem, I'm sure.

Sunday, December 6

Today I'm trying not to use my cane much. I think self-confidence is a big part of it. Yesterday I wrote my first note to my mother. I can't wait until she sees me all better again.

Monday, December 7

This morning David called me from school to tell me that he had made the basketball team. I wasn't surprised. Treatment #9. Only eight more to go after that. Feeling a bit stronger every day. Come Spring, this will all be a dream— or a nightmare!!

Tuesday, December 8

Treatment #10. Still haven't lost any hair yet, but if it happens, it happens. Just trying to finish up some bills.

Wednesday, December 9

Treatment #11. So, far, I still have my hair. Got rid of my eye patch and the bed in the family room.

Thursday, December 10

Treatment #12. I didn't sleep well last night. I think I am starting to lose my hair!!! I have a hard time looking down, and also, writing. Things are blurry and I'm still uncoordinated, but I'm getting there.

Friday, December 11

Treatment # 13. Had a bad night last night. I'm upset about losing my hair. I suppose this should be the least of my worries. Am working hard every day.

Saturday, December 12

No treatment today. Yeah! I *really* am losing my hair!!! There is a baby squirrel loose in the house. Today we're getting our Christmas tree.

Sunday, December 13

Got all my cotton square scarves together. Think I am going to need them. Today we'll decorate the tree.

Monday, December 14

Treatment #14. Only three more. It's such a strain writing in this journal, because my hand doesn't want to go fast enough, and everything is blurry.

Tuesday, December 15

Treatment #15. Only two more to go after today. Yesterday I played pool with David; I think I beat him!

Wednesday, December 16

Treatment #16. Only one more to go. Yesterday, I was a little more wobbly than usual. I think I am getting tired of this whole thing. My scalp hurts.

Thursday, December 17

Treatment #17. My last one! Hurray!!! I'm wearing a Santa Claus hat today. Dressed in red and green. Peter went to school late today. Also, lost his basketball game to Wilmington. I don't think he got a chance to play.

Friday, December 18

Treatments done. Time to "veg-out." Didn't lose as much hair as I thought. David is giving a Christmas party with Leslie, Aubrey's daughter. It's hard to write.

Saturday, December 19

Woke up with a headache this morning. Could it be because of two hours of *The Sound of Music* last night on TV, or maybe I'm starting my period? Peter left me a note, telling me he had a flat tire. Something else to take care of. Acton-Boxborough beat Weston (#1 team in Division 2) in OT last night.

Sunday, December 20

It's snowing today. Judy is here. Think it's going to be kind of a lazy day.

Monday December 21

Second day of my period. I guess that's a good sign, but I thought radiation would cause some delay.

Tuesday, December 22

It's sunny out today. Nothing much to say. Just trying to recoup. Would write a lot more (and I'm sure better) if I could see. Things are blurry.

Wednesday, December 23

Only two more days until Christmas. My cleaning lady made me a doily, designed into a circular wooden frame, and now it is hanging in my bedroom window.

Thursday, December 24

'Twas the night before Christmas…Dr. Vaillant is coming today. So is Kathy, my visiting physical therapist. I'll just mention again that I could write better if I could see better. Things are coming, but ever so slowly.

Friday, December 25

It's Christmas Day. Friends brought a lot of nice presents. It's a good day, but now want to get on to 1988, and feeling better. Peter is out with his friend giving out free candy canes. David is at Don's house, probably talking about their Christmas presents. I've noticed that I am writing too fast, at the same time, squinting less. Both eyes are open.

Saturday, December 26

'Twas the day after Christmas, and oh, what a mess! We had a good day yesterday. The family called. My friend, Julene, came to visit. I had not seen her in a couple years. Peter is going to his father's house today, and overnight. I think he needs a break from me. David will probably go next weekend. I think he needs a break from me, too.

Sunday, December 27

Last night the furnace broke, and we had no heat. The man came, and now the heat is on. Judy is here and we are chatting away.

Monday, December 28

Minuteman Ridge did their caroling last night. Next year I'll be with them. Believe it or not, Peter played golf today!

Tuesday, December 29

It's snowing out today. Maybe 4-7 inches possible. I made an appointment to see Dr. Hochberg on January 12. Just love going to the Mass General Zoo!

Wednesday, December 30

It's really cold today. Maybe a wind chill factor of 20 degrees below zero. There are people out there who don't think I am going to make it, but I already have, and I am getting better every day. Perhaps I AM A MIRACLE!

Thursday, December 31

It's New Year's Eve. Maybe I'll get dressed up tonight, and knock a few socks off! Cleaning up some clutter around here. Getting ready for 1988. Mom says 1988 rhymes with GREAT. I think she's right!

10.

HAPPY NEW YEAR

Friday, January 1, 1988

Happy New Year! Feeling a bit stronger every day. Going to start physical therapy on an outpatient basis. Peter and Joel, Aubrey's son, are driving David to the bus station today. He's going to his father's house. I DID get dressed up last night. Rhinestone earrings and shoes. Slow danced in my sneakers with Aubrey. Had a few sips of champagne. I am going to be an example for many people this year. I am strong and my mind is set.

Saturday, January 2

Today, while standing, I touched my toes and put my hands flat on the floor, without bending my knees. Would love to show Drs. Hochberg and Gibai this one. Donna is coming again today to help take my clothes upstairs. Yesterday she took down the tree, and cleaned up the family room. What would I do without her? Glad to see the holidays come to an end. Every day a little bit better.

Sunday, January 3

Last night I looked at the back of my head with a mirror. I was shocked and pretty upset. I guess I didn't think I had lost *that* much hair! David's coming back from his father's house in Connecticut today.

Monday, January 4

Not much going on today. It snowed, and school was delayed one hour. Since this was the first day back from vacation, the kids loved it! As usual though, all other schools were closed.

Tuesday, January 5

It's bitter cold outside today. I may take a ride to the bank. On the other hand, maybe I'll send someone. I may try to make some chocolate chip cookies.

Wednesday, January 6

I went down to the basement today for the first time in over six months. I was the only one in the house. Pretty messy, but not bad under the circumstances. Still bitter outside.

Thursday, January 7

I'm trying to do something new every day. I may try to attend the fourth quarter of David's Acton-Concord basketball game. But then again, it may be better to attend a recreation game on Saturday first—less people, less noise, less action.

Friday, January 8

I didn't go to David's game, but I saw the video. They won. David looked good, even though he fouled out. Poor "reffing." of course! Peter did groceries after basketball practice. He has a lot to handle. My right leg felt a little lighter yesterday. I actually feel a little pretty today.

Saturday, January 9

It really snowed last night. David is going with his father and the rest of the team (with their fathers) to a Northeastern University basketball game today. I never know what each day is going to bring. I continually surprise myself with little improvements. People come in and out all day long. I wish I didn't have such a hard time writing, but that will come.

Sunday, January 10

Yesterday I felt sort of "itchy." Jimmy, my brother, called last night, and told me I should get out. I'm planning on going to Lynn's house across the street. I haven't been anywhere except for hospitals, and out for a few rides, for months. Kind of scary getting out.

Monday, January 11

Today I'm going to Joyce's house, just a few houses down from me. Need to keep getting out. Tomorrow is the clinic with Dr. Hochberg et al at Mass General. I can't wait to show them what I can do.

Tuesday, January 12

Today I went to Mass General, and showed off in front of Drs. Bashir and Levine from radiation. I touched my toes, and they said, "When you fall, which way do you fall?" I said, "I DON'T FALL!" I walked with my cane from the examination room in the Cox Building to the front door (long walk). I have to have a CAT Scan and go back in a month. The doctors were impressed and delighted with my progress, and I felt good about myself (no glasses).

Wednesday, January 13

Today I will try to go to part of David's practice. I need to see what it feels like to enter the gym, and deal with the lights, action and noise.

Thursday, January 14

Today is Aubrey's birthday. I sent a Japanese-style flower arrangement to his office. I'll go to the fourth quarter of David's basketball game today. Yesterday I took the trash out, and took a walk down to the mailbox (with some help).

Friday, January 15

We're having a heat wave today; it might get to 20 degrees! My cleaning lady just informed me that she is going on vacation two weeks in February. I wonder how we'll do.

Saturday, January 16

This morning I went to David's recreation basketball game. They won. I've been working on a jigsaw puzzle. Not my favorite thing to do, but it's become a big part of my day.

Sunday, January 17

Peter left early this morning to go skiing at Mt. Sunapee, New Hampshire. I started my period yesterday. Slept in late today, and had to deal with a messy bed.

Monday, January 18

I had to back the car over Boswell's (Isn't that a great name for a dog?) line today and yesterday. It will be a while before my coordination is back. David just left for Boston with friends.

Tuesday, January 19

Yesterday Peter and I cleaned the garage. Today I am going to *walk* into the bank, and go to part of Peter's basketball game.

Wednesday, January 20

Today I am going to see Dr. Vinger, the ophthalmologist. He saw me in the hospital when I was in Intensive Care. It will be interesting to see if he is going to prescribe something, or if he wants my eyes to stabilize a bit more.

Thursday, January 21

Well, I have to get bifocals. No permanent damage. That's what they told me at Mass Eye and Ear, when I was at Mass General having chemo. Only old age. It will be good to see again. Today I'm going to try to go to David's whole game.

Friday, January 22

Not much to say. Pam, my visiting nurse, is coming this morning. I'm trying to do some dancing to relax myself. I'm too stiff when I write and when I walk.

Saturday, January 23

Lynn is here brushing Boswell. So far nothing planned for today. Slept in late.

Sunday, January 24

Today I'm planning on taking a little walk outside. It's about 35 degrees. Nothing new and exciting. My jigsaw puzzle is coming along. Walked down Captain Brown's Lane, my street, as far as Quigley's house, with Aubrey.

Monday, January 25

Going to get my glasses today. Can't wait. Every little thing helps. Upon leaving the optical shop, I noticed an elderly woman with a cane; I had mine also. We shared stories. She had a cancer story, too. I said, "I had brain cancer, but it is all gone." She said, "Don't be too sure of that, dearie!" Thanks a lot. She really made my day! The sympathetic part in me said, "Poor thing. She must be a miserable and bitter old woman." The other part of me, the angry part, said, "How dare you?"

Tuesday, January 26

Today I see Dr. Moore. It's been exactly five months since the biopsy. Good news from Dr. Moore. He thinks I'm doing fantastic!

Wednesday, January 27

Maggie, an old friend from my earlier days in Boston, is coming today. She said something about giving me a facial. This will be the first time I have seen her in a while.

Thursday, January 28

Today I'm going to David's basketball game. I've been busy and active the past two days, so I think I will relax a lot today.

Friday January 29

Last night I was upset, because even though the doctors are delighted, I'm getting tired of all of this. I want to be "normal." I want to walk right and write right. I want my coordination back!

Saturday, January 30

This morning I went to David's basketball game, and this afternoon I walked around the block with Aubrey.

Sunday, January 31

Last day of January. Hurray! Will walk around the block today. One more feather.

11.

CANCER-FREE

Monday, February 1

Yeah February! A little bit closer to spring. Today I have a CAT Scan, and I'm a little scared, naturally. But last week Dr. Moore said that he didn't think they would find anything. Let's hope.

Tuesday, February 2

The groundhog did not see its shadow, so maybe spring will come early. Hope! Hope!

Wednesday, February 3

Nothing much happening today. I may make some cookies. My left eye is twitching.

Thursday, February 4

It's really snowy outside. I walked around the block yesterday, but it looks like today is out. Dr. Vaillant is supposed to come today, but it's pretty bad out there. (He came.) Yesterday he gave me good news about my CAT Scan.

Friday, February 5

Dr. V. said my progress is better and faster then he ever hoped or expected, and that the rest of me would come together like costumes, set, lights, etc. for a show. He knows I performed in the community theater. I am CANCER-FREE!

Saturday, February 6

Today the electrologist is coming. I am either removing it from my face or trying to grow it on my head!

Sunday, February 7

I am going to iron a shirt today. Maybe I will go to Nancy's house to meet Anita, her friend who has Multiple Sclerosis. I try to dance a little every day.

Monday, February 8

Today I am going to Nancy's house. I seem to be incredibly busy every day.

Tuesday, February 9

Went to Mass General to see the doctors. They think I am doing super! Peter played a great basketball game today. He made 16 points, sunk a three-pointer, and hit numerous shots from the foul line. Both teams, the varsity and junior varsity beat undefeated Lincoln-Sudbury. The junior varsity went into OT, and won by one point in the last two seconds. My poor heart!

Wednesday, February 10

I'm going for a walk with Kay, a neighbor who lives behind me. Nothing really scheduled today.

Thursday, February 11

I did three big things today. I started physical therapy. (We're going to work on balance.) I went out to the Mail Coach Restaurant with Lynn. (First time out to eat in months. Piece of cake!) I went to David's last basketball game. They won against Concord.

Friday, February 12

No school today. It is snowing really hard. David is sick.

Saturday, February 13

David was sick last night. I got him some medicine at 4 a.m., and, to my surprise, he crawled into bed with me. He must have been sleepwalking or disoriented, because this is not a usual occurrence. I asked him, "David, is everything OK?" He said, "Yes," and then promptly got up and went to his own room. I wonder if he just felt secure being near me because of everything that has been happening to me. Nothing exciting is planned for today, but that does not mean nothing exciting will happen.

Sunday, February 14

It's Valentine's Day. I am giving Aubrey some red socks.

Monday, February 15

Physical Therapy (PT). With the exercises they gave me, I should have the cutest butt east of the Mississippi!

Tuesday, February 16

I did my new exercises this morning. I can tell already that they are going to work. I'm going to walk much better.

Wednesday, February 17

Third day of my period. For some reason I have cramps.

Thursday, February 18

Yesterday I walked around the block with my cane by myself! Yeah! Last night I had pains in the back of my head, and today I have a cold. Am waiting on calls from Drs.Vaillant and Moore.

Friday, February 19

PT today. I have the flu. That's all I need. My visiting nurse, Pam, is coming today for the last time. She took a blood sample when she was here, confirming the flu. She and I may go for a walk. We did.

Saturday, February 20

Sick today. Didn't get dressed.

Sunday, February 21

Still sick. I fit into my jeans!

Monday, February 22

Still sick and stuffed up.

Tuesday, February 23

Still miserable. Getting better.

Wednesday, February 24

Getting better. I think my hair is starting to come in.

Thursday, February 25

Tonight is Peter's basketball banquet. I don't know if I will be able to go or not. Did not go. Not well enough from the flu.

Friday, February 26

Today marks six months since my surgery. Still feeling lousy from the flu. Don't know if I will go to PT today. Did not go.

Saturday, February 27

Went around the block alone with my cane. In skating competition, Debbie Thomas loses to Katerina Witt.

Sunday, February 28

Walked down the street with no cane. Amazing grace! Took Aubrey's arm the rest of the way. He just got back from skiing at Sugarloaf. Missed him.

Monday, February 29

Last day of the month. Looking forward to March. Going to David's basketball banquet tonight. Sat with Aubrey in the very back of the room on folding chairs next to the vending machine. Easier than being in the midst of the crowd as I was still uncomfortable with my unsteadiness. Moved forward to talk to the coach after the crowd dispersed.

12.

GETTING BACK IN THE SWING

Tuesday, March 1

Yeah March! Went to PT. They said I didn't lose a bit being out with the flu last week. Am starting to wear leotards and tights. Might as well get into it with a spirit! Walked around the block alone carrying my cane.

Wednesday, March 2

Errands today, plus usual exercise routines.

Thursday, March 3

Am going to the dentist today. Hope it doesn't snow this weekend—cramps my style!!

Friday, March 4

Some snow, but it won't last. Cleaning lady back today. Yeah!

Saturday, March 5

I'm starting to walk a little better. Yesterday in PT they told me to squeeze my buttocks 'til it burns. I said, "I can tell this is going to be a fun class!"

Sunday, March 6

David is having pancakes next to me. Boswell is barking outside. Nothing really exciting to report, except I think I'm walking better.

Monday, March 7

Believe it or not, I walked 1.2 miles yesterday. Did it again today.

Tuesday, March 8

Today I'll vote for Dukakis. Getting new glasses. 1.2 miles again.

Wednesday, March 9

Dukakis and Bush win big.

Thursday, March 10

Nothing big scheduled for today.

Friday, March 11

Yesterday I threaded a needle on the first try, and sewed a button on my sweater.

Saturday, March 12

Time marches on. Will probably go to David's last recreation game. It's nice outside—may reach 50 degrees.

Sunday, March 13

Yesterday I went to Quill and Press (stationery store) with Donna to buy some birthday and Easter stuff—$61. Also, went to the Triple A market with Aubrey. First day I had been to any store for months!!

Monday, March 14

Yesterday I went to the Purity Supreme supermarket and to the bookstore next door with Aubrey. It's snowing. Ugh!

Tuesday, March 15

Am getting my new glasses today. Split my bifocals because they made me dizzier than I already am. Made them into two pairs of glasses, one for reading; the other for distance. Started my period yesterday. It snowed a little. Everything is wonderful. Ugh!

Wednesday, March 16

College night at the high school. I hemmed a dress yesterday. Did a good job. Have been taking Vitamin C like crazy. David has his cold again.

Thursday, March 17

Happy St. Patrick's Day! My tax man is coming today. The sun is shining, and it's windy.

Friday, March 18

Went to J & S Sports, and also The Outdoor Store in Maynard yesterday. Am sick of being sick.

Saturday, March 19

Peter has SAT today. Going to see Lynn Hughes Trio tonight. She is my friend. Loved going, but very hard on my eyes.

Sunday, March 20

Peter's birthday. He is 17 years old. He really liked his portable phone I bought him. Went to David's game in Bedford. Before I sat in a folding chair on the side because I didn't have the balance to sit on the bleacher seats. Sat in the bleachers with everyone else today. Lost to Sudbury by two points.

Monday, March 21

CAT Scan today. Not looking forward to it.

Tuesday, March 22

No news yet on CAT Scan. Doing errands. 7 p.m.—CAT Scan is good.

Wednesday, March 23

Am calling Occupational Therapy for fine motor coordination.

Thursday, March 24

Raked leaves today.

Friday, March 25

Furnace gets cleaned, if he can find it in all the mess. Peter goes to his father's house. David plays in championship basketball game against Sudbury. A-B won.

Saturday, March 26

David's going into Boston with friends on the train. Today marks seven months since the surgery. Went to Marshall's. Bought some sheets.

Sunday, March 27

Went to the mall. Bought David sneakers. Did pretty well, except ran into a few clothes racks.

Monday, March 28

Getting stronger. Stopped by to see my travel agent to straighten out some business. Stopped at Kathy's house.

Tuesday, March 29

Mass General today. They said my progress was so good that I was getting "boring". Bought a pouch-type handbag. Had a hot fudge sundae at Friendly's with Aubrey. Walked 1.2 miles, no cane. Talked to neighbors. Nice day.

Wednesday, March 30

Did laundry. Raked leaves.

Thursday, March 31

OT (occupational therapy) evaluation at Emerson Hospital with Pat White. I hold my pen too tightly. Strength is 60 lbs. (squeeze) on the right side, and 58 lbs. on the left. She gave me a bunch of things to do. Definitely need it.

Friday, April 1

Good Friday and April Fool's Day. David played his regular "spray" trick on me (taping sprayer on kitchen sink with black tape, so that water sprays when you open faucet). Every year my kids do it, and every year I forget. Sometimes I used the same trick on them by leaving the tape on. They would forget when they had to wash their hands or get a drink of water. Then they would get sprayed. David went golfing today. Yucko writing! (frustrated with my writing)

Saturday April 2

Raked leaves. Fixed ham for tomorrow. Going to Aubrey's house for Easter.

Sunday, April 3

Easter at Aubrey's. I cooked the ham. He did the rest. Pink roses, candles, linen tablecloth and napkins. David had to wash some windows at Aubrey's because he lost a bet with him.

Monday, April 4

Stamps went up to 25 cents from 22 cents. Did some shopping, voted; went to the bank.

Tuesday, April 5

Raked leaves. Did laundry. Cleaned house. Made hamburgers.

Wednesday, April 6

Will rake leaves. Who knows what else? I'm always trying something, and someone is always dropping in. Peter is trying out for tennis; David, for baseball.

Thursday, April 7

Actually cleaned out the shop and swept out the laundry room in the basement. Cleaned out the kitchen cupboards the other day.

Friday April 8

Took down all the drapes. Must have the spring cleaning bug. The more I do, the more independent I become and the better I feel. Still have the numb feeling in the mouth area at times. Still ataxia. Am getting better, but never fast enough.

Saturday, April 9

Went to David's first soccer game. 0–0. He quit baseball tryouts. Peter got a ticket and backstage pass to Stevie Ray Vaughan concert.

Sunday, April 10

Been doing a lot of cleaning, but took time out to sit in the sun with some neighbors.

Monday, April 11

Just more cleaning today. Am going to a meeting tonight for David's Washington, D.C. trip.

Tuesday, April 12

Started my period this morning. Ever since my treatments, it has been coming every 28 days.

Wednesday, April 13

Sent out tax forms. Getting ready for window washers tomorrow.

Thursday, April 14

Window washers today. I did a lot of wood cleaning, laundry and sewing.

Friday, April 15

Taxes due. Ours are all in. Had to pay out this time. Ridiculous! But, it's been a funny year. Helping David get ready for Washington, D.C. Decided to have cleaning lady every other week, instead of every week.

Saturday, April 16

I woke up around 3 a.m. Then Boswell came upstairs around 4:30 a.m. and David left for Washington D.C., with his friend, Drew, and about 58 others at 5:45 a.m. So far, it's been a busy day!

Sunday, April 17

Today David and Drew were selected to put the wreath on the unknown soldier's grave with the changing of the guard in a ceremony in Washington D.C. I cleaned out the fireplace.

Monday, April 18

Yesterday I did 20 full push-ups. Boswell's birthday, 10 years old. Peter went to the Red Sox game. David got back from Washington D.C. Boston Marathon—Hussein and Rosa Moto. I wrapped pennies.

Tuesday, April 19

Peter just informed me that he is going to the Junior-Senior Prom, with Jenny, a sophomore.

Wednesday, April 20

I got frustrated and cried at PT. Things never move fast enough. I work hard, but I am impatient. I want to drive a car. Keep dreamin'.

Thursday, April 21

Peter leaves for New York with a friend. I have the stomach flu. Vomited twice.

Friday, April 22

Still weak. Aubrey's back from Puerto Rico.

Saturday, April 23

Went to David's soccer game. It rained. They lost 1–0.

Sunday, April 24

Today we received our last meal from friends. Everyone has been so kind, but it is good to be on my own again. It's 9:10 p.m., and I finished proofreading a 13-page paper for Peter. Felt good.

Monday, April 25

I baked an apple pie. Mom called. She's coming on the 30th.

Tuesday, April 26

I saw Dr. Moore, my neurologist, today. He said my improvement was "striking". I see him again in four months.

Wednesday, April 27

Stopped wearing scarves on my head a few days ago. Raked leaves. Walked.

Thursday, April 28

OT. My therapist was extremely impressed with my progress since last month. She suggested I do video games, and try the car out in a parking lot. Scary!

Friday, April 29

PT. Aubrey took me and observed. Then we had lunch. Linguine with garlic and olive oil. My sister Linda's birthday. Peter rented his tux for the prom.

13.

"TIE A YELLOW RIBBON 'ROUND THE OLD OAK TREE"

Saturday, April 30

Have to rest today. Going to meet Mom at the airport. Can't wait to see her, and will she be surprised! (She said, "Don't wait up. I'll wake you when I get home.") She was surprised. Met her with a dozen yellow roses, her favorite. Tied a yellow ribbon around my old oak tree in front of my house.

Sunday, May 1

Rested today. So good to see Mom.

Monday, May 2

PT. Mom watched. Went grocery shopping. Cooked a turkey. Wasn't too good.

Tuesday, May 3

Peter got inducted into the National Honor Society. He was all dressed up in a sports jacket, but I noticed he chose not to wear socks! Mom and I were so proud of him. Mom and I (mostly Mom) made stuffed grape leaves and kibbee.

Wednesday, May 4

I felt improvement today. I'm walking better or something. Did 20 full pushups again.

Thursday, May 5

Pat, my occupational therapist, asked me if I tried driving in a parking lot. She said I could do more than I think I can. Maybe this week. I walked down the junior high path, across from my house that leads to the school. Pleasant wooded area.

Friday, May 6

PT. Balance on one foot improving. I put on my panties standing up! Starting to play video games per OT. Hate it.

Saturday, May 7

Went with Mom to see "Carousel" at Theatre III, the community theater where I performed in approximately 17 shows. It was great to see all my friends. I felt so special, even though I had barely any hair. The cast gave me an autographed poster which I will cherish forever.

Sunday, May 8

Mother's Day. David got me a rose. Peter made me a card. It was special having my Mom here. I made a scallop and linguine dinner, and baked two large apple pies. Candles and linen. Silver and china. I drove today for the first time in eleven months. It was scary. Drove in the junior high school parking lot, and then home via Hayward Road. It must have felt strange for Peter riding in the passenger seat—I know it was for me!!

Monday, May 9

Muxie, long time friend of the family, came for a visit. I see Dr. V. at his office. We compared my handwriting (signature) with a day in November. Huge improvement!

Tuesday, May 10

Called Dr.V. about small lump on head. False alarm. Just a sebaceous cyst. Thank goodness!

Wednesday, May 11

PT. Did 25 pushups at home.

Thursday, May 12

OT. Played catch with a large ball and a tennis ball. Felt like an awkward little kid. Muxie's last night here. Sure was good to see him. Peter and David enjoyed him. Mom sparkled. Walked at least 1.5 miles today. Went onto the wooded path leading to the junior high school.

Friday, May 13

Going to the Rockport shoe outlet in Marlboro to buy some shoes.

Saturday, May 14

Boswell bit Matt, Peter's friend. No stitches, but still very upsetting. Prom night. Peter looked handsome and very grown up in his tux. I met Jenny, his date. She wore a pink dress and looked very sweet. Took a lot of pictures.

Sunday, May 15

Prom continued to the beach. David and I washed the car, and I drove around our neighborhood, Minuteman Ridge. Reflex and coordination have a long way to go.

Monday, May 16

Going to Valerie's house for lunch with Mom. Cooking lobsters tonight. Mom leaves tomorrow for California.

Tuesday, May 17

Mom leaves. Sad day. She's my best friend. Cried at PT.

14.

ON MY OWN AGAIN

Wednesday, May 18

Went to Quill and Press again. Found out I did not have extension for PT. Need to appeal.

Thursday, May 19

Today I typed a letter to Harvard Community Health Plan, my health insurance company, on the Apple IIc computer. Slowly, but I did it. Ordered a bike and stabilizers from Lincoln Guide Service, $686, including accessories. I deserve it.

Friday May 20

Am slowly improving. Wrote a letter to Petra, my travel agent, on my computer.

Saturday, May 21

Went to David's soccer game.

Sunday, May 22

Bounced/dribbled the ball 54 times. Cleaned my room. Organized my clothes. The Celtics beat the Hawks today in Game #7.

Monday, May 23

Called nutritionist to see if I should cut back on vitamin dosage. Bounced/dribbled the ball 90 times! Hot outside.

Tuesday, May 24

Laundry. Cleaning. Hot again. Thunderstorm. Bounced the ball 155 times!

Wednesday, May 25

The painters were here. They took up a lot of space, so I had a hard time today. Rainy and raw. Went out to lunch with a friend. That was fun.

Thursday, May 26

OT. Dribbled the ball about 200 times! Pat said that pretty soon they will be running out of things for me to do.

Friday, May 27

Am learning how to hop and run. Really feel stupid.

Saturday, May 28

Am noticing slight improvement in my eyes. When I'm walking, I can look out a little further, instead of down near my feet. Am starting to practice heel-to-toe walking. The neighborhood pool opened.

Sunday, May 29

Today Peter and David drove to Connecticut to see their father. This is the first time. I was worried about Peter, and he was concerned about leaving me alone. We'll both do all right.

Monday, May 30

Today I jogged about 100 yards. Looked pretty silly, but I did it. Peter and David made it back OK. No problem.

Tuesday, May 31

I want to start on my book. Had CAT Scan.

Wednesday, June 1

My sister Georgia's birthday. Did various shopping. Celtics lost to the Pistons. I drove the car again. Feels better.

Thursday, June 2

OT. Pat said that I was doing some of the most difficult activities they have. She said I performed better than most "normal" people. I said I thought my problem was that I performed better than I really was. Jogged 300-400 yards today. Hard for me to tell.

Friday, June 3

Going to pick up my bike today in Kay's pick-up truck. Got myself some wheels. David sees Dr. Blute about his weak ankles (I had a flat tire. We never got there.) Katie O'Grady's graduation party. CAT Scan is clean.

Saturday, June 4

Bike didn't work out. It was a great idea using a regular bike, and adding stabilizers, but I was off balance, and it was too hard to steer. Then Aubrey and I went to Allerton Bike Shop in Hull and bought a beautiful blue trike.

Sunday, June 5

At first, I couldn't ride the trike, and I felt humiliated. But before you knew it, I was zooming all over. The neighborhood kids thought it was pretty cool, and so did the adults. Five-year-old Sean had a horn on his tricycle just like mine, and wanted to race me down the street. I can't remember the last time I had such a feeling of freedom and control. Today I skipped. Both Peter and David have bad colds. I'm going to tutor Jeffrey, Donna's son, tomorrow night. Really excited about this! Went to a neighbor, Al's 50th birthday party on my new trike. Wore my white jumpsuit, white stockings, white shoes. It's fun to dress up again. I encouraged my friend, Anita, to ride my trike, and I showed her some exercises on her family room floor. It's a banner day!

Monday, June 6

Jeffrey didn't show. Peter's Dad got him a 1976 BMW. Rode my trike. Love it!

15.

THE FIRST DAY OF THE REST OF MY LIFE

Tuesday, June 7

Started my period. Seems like it's always a big deal! Went to Mass General. Saw Dr. Bashir and Joyce Jandl, R.N. They were extremely pleased with my progress, and had me do my traditional walk around the examining table. Also, saw Dr. Pruitt in the hall. Hadn't seen her since chemo days. She was surprised, and said she knew how well I was doing, because Dr. Moore sends her reports. Also, ran into Dr. Lingood. She's British. (If only she knew we called her "Fergie"). Then Aubrey and I went upstairs to Baker 5 to see if any of my old nurses were there. We saw Joan, one of my favorites, and she just about dropped her teeth. I was dressed in that same white jumpsuit with white stockings. Then we went out to lunch at the Willow Pond Restaurant in Concord, and had a wonderful clam dinner. I tutored Jeffrey. I think he has a lot of potential. I know how to "do" kids.

Wednesday, June 8

Nothing exciting planned for today. Laundry and cooking and cleaning. Maybe I'll try getting some of this stuff on the computer. It's a nice day, so I'll get some sun.

Thursday, June 9

OT. Pat thinks I'm ready to go back to work. I know when I'll be ready. This body and this mind will know. I'll never do anything I don't want to do again.

Friday, June 10

PT. Doing well. Improving. Eighth grade dance. A big deal. David's wearing a black leather tie. He's kind of going with Debbie. He's meeting her at the school. Took Boswell to the vet. He has a bleeding cyst.

Saturday, June 11

The kids left on the bus to Connecticut to pick up Peter's car. I bought him some jumper cables, a med kit, and a bunch of other stuff. I spent a few hours at my neighborhood pool, and did a lot of yapping. I bought a mini-trampoline. Aubrey had me over for dinner. We had steak and French fries and salad.

Sunday, June 12

Peter brought his car home. 1976 BMW 2002. Black. Tan interior. Real classy. Actually got into the pool. Wore my bikini.

Monday, June 13

Today is the first day of the rest of my life. I went to my friend, Judy York's third grade class, at St. Bridget's School in Maynard. They have been praying for me all year, and I wanted to see them. I showed them before and after photos, my journals, and my Theraplast (similar to putty for exercising hands). We took some photos, which I will copy and send to them: Kate, Meghan, Steve, Garrett, Bobby and Bill. I gave them each a yellow carnation, and they each made me a huge get well card. They asked if they were going to be in my book. A very exciting morning, but I didn't cry, as I usually do when I am filled with emotion.

Tuesday. June 14

Walking better. Hot today. Mid-90's. Pistons beat Lakers. It's all tied up.

Wednesday June 15

Hot again. May reach 98 degrees. Maybe I'll try to get into the pool today. Maybe I'll wear my white bikini. I love showing off because I work so hard.

Thursday, June 16

Took David to see Dr. Blute for his ankles. Injury from sports, especially mounting and dismounting in gymnastics, and also flat feet. The pharmacist asked whether I would be performing my traditional Middle Eastern dance at the Acton-Boxborough Jamboree this summer. I always appear to be better than I really am.

Friday. June 17

The first cool day we've had for a while.

Saturday. June 18

David's last soccer game. Pool party. I'm selling tickets for eats and drinks for an hour. They'll just have to line up, and wait for me while I struggle to make change. I keep trying to do different things.

Sunday, June 19

Father's Day. Joel, Peter's friend, made a seafood dinner for his dad, Aubrey, and invited us. Peter helped him cook. (Ed, my kids' father, is in France.) Had another one of those "spells" where I wish I was "normal." so I could go to the movies and do other fun things. Went to church with Lynn to hear the music. Put a dress on for the first time in a year. Wore my favorite white one, with ruffles at the hips, white patterned stockings and white shoes. I just love white in the summer.

Monday, June 20

Went to my friend, Elizabeth's house, for lunch in Carlisle. We did some catching up. Jeffrey came to my house for tutoring. He had to be convinced to come during the summer months, if only for once a week.

Tuesday, June 21

PT. I balanced on my left foot for over a minute, and my right foot for 44 seconds. Peter is in the middle of exams. It's math today. David's at Whalom Park with his friends.

Wednesday, June 22

Last exam for Peter. Last day of school. When school started I was in intensive care at the hospital, and now it is the last day of school. Peter is going to the beach with friends.

16.

LIFE IN THE FAST LANE

Thursday, June 23

Peter had an accident while driving my car. He was making a left turn, and hit a car with a priest and some altar boys from Sudbury. Everyone was OK, but my car was totaled. Tonight the priest called me. He said that I should be proud of Peter. He said Peter was truly concerned, and that he handled the situation well. He also said that he was the most polite young man he had ever met.

Friday, June 24

Peter went to Nautilus. David did some yard work for a neighbor. They went to the dentist. I baked a birthday cake for David.

Saturday, June 25

David's birthday—14 years old. He was at the Fifer's Festival in Boxborough with his friend, Michael, all day, and Peter was at a barbecue. It seems as though there is always a lot of keeping track of people.

Sunday, June 26

Nothing on the calendar today. Might do some ironing. That's what I get for liking cotton so much.

Monday, June 27

Went looking at rugs today with Donna. I like wool, the best—and most expensive. I didn't get anything. Bought some leg warmers for 99 cents and a zipper for 10 cents at Building #19.

Tuesday, June 28

PT. I'm learning to walk better. I can feel it. Jane Loureiro, my therapist, walked behind me, putting resistance with stretchy fabric to my right thigh, gradually lessening. Whenever I walk, I think of what she termed the "phantom hand," (the stretchy fabric as a hand) and it feels more right. Had lunch with Aubrey. Ate outside, European-style. It was nice.

Wednesday, June 29

Found out my car is totaled. Motor and suspension are damaged. Too bad, it was a nice car. But, "c'est la vie." At least no one got hurt. I'm sad, but not mad. Nothing is that important. I'm already starting to look around for another car. It's funny how your priorities change. David went to the Red Sox game. Peter went swimming in a pond at a friend's house. He likes doing that.

Thursday, June 30

David got his braces on his lower teeth. We say goodbye to the car, and get the license plate, etc.

Friday, July 1

Went to a car dealer to look for a new car.

Saturday, July 2

Went to see the car at the dealer again, this time with the kids and Aubrey. I took it around the parking lot, and Peter took it for a serious drive test. Sort of torn. I am not doing any driving yet, just parking lots. On the other hand, if I don't get it, I won't have something to jump into when I am ready. And I'll procrastinate and get more and more afraid. Oh yeah, Peter lost his second and only set of car keys at Nautilus, and sent me into a tailspin. We ended up finding both sets of keys. When we got home, David said, "Mom, are we going to be in your book?" I said, "Yes, under a chapter titled STRESS!!!"

Sunday, July 3

Peter and his friends are "jamming" upstairs. Two guys on guitars and Peter on his drums. The other night there were three guitars. They actually sound pretty good. Loud, but good! I like to practice skipping and running on the path through the woods. It's private, and nobody can see me.

Monday, July 4

Fourth of July. My brother Jim's birthday. He is in Sweden and Norway giving a paper. He is a professor of animal science at the University of California in Davis. Spent most of the day with the Valades and their family and friends. Walked down through the woods to watch the fireworks at the high school area. I was surprised how much easier it's becoming to get up and down from the blanket. Too sick to go last year. Problem focusing, but better.

Tuesday, July 5

I am running faster and more naturally through the woods. It feels good when "I find the right place," the right feeling in my body and mind.

Wednesday, July 6

I did some comparison shopping and went to another Mazda dealer. Bought a car. "Will you work with us on these prices?" "No, I will not. I know what you paid for the car." "You mean you want this car at the dealer's price?" "Yes, I do." Got a great deal. Slightly over cost. If they can play the game, so can I. My therapist had given me some pointers on buying a car.

Thursday, July 7

Did tutoring today. I'm a good teacher because I'm sensitive to kids and aware of their needs.

Friday, July 8

Peter went white water rafting. I feel like I'm walking better. Climbed up the basement steps without holding on to the railing. Used the Biodex machine at physical therapy. M's are hard to write.

Saturday, July 9

Last night there was thunder and lightning. Boswell kept me up all night. David went to his father's house today. Aubrey drove us to the bus station. He's so reliable and so kind, and always there. Today I got into the pool. The water was warm. I was able to walk and jump without holding on to the side of the pool. Now, I can do exercises, and work on strengthening and balancing. I'm so proud of myself. What a feeling!

Sunday, July 10

Hot today. Spent most of my time at the pool. Did some running around and some exercises. I love it when the water is that warm.

Monday, July 11

Might reach 100 degrees. May walk to the post office. Climbed the junior high school steps. No railing.

Tuesday, July 12

PT. Used the ankle board without holding on to anything. When I got home, I continued to work out in the pool for two hours. Did a lot of yakking, too.

Wednesday, July 13

Domestic chores always. Minuteman Ridge swim meet. My kids quit competing two or three years ago. They have other sports and activities they would rather do. Peter's been doing a lot of "jamming". It amazes me how well he and his three friends "play off" of each other. I'm walking better. I think about the "phantom hand" giving resistance on my right side. I also concentrate in walking in the center of my right foot. Feels good. Feels right.

Thursday, July 14

OT. I was wondering if I could go to California in December. My therapist thinks I can fly in a plane right NOW. She thinks I need to work more on my confidence. It's easy to lose a lot of confidence when you're going through an ordeal. Funny how brain cancer can take it right out of you. Jim called. He's back from Sweden.

Friday, July 15

Did more pool therapy.

17.

NEVER A DULL MOMENT

Saturday, July 16

My area code in Massachusetts changed to 508. A small sparrow flew into the house, just as my financial advisor was arriving. He trapped it in a kitchen towel, and then set it free. Never a dull moment. Baked an apple pie. Tonight I took the big step and went DANCING! First time in over a year. It was fun, but my balance, my right side, has a way to go. Plus I'm still dizzy. I wasn't my usual kicky self. Felt like I had bubble gum stuck on the sole of my right shoe. Same as everything else, my mind is racing away, but my body can't catch up. Went with Aubrey. He is the only one who would understand at this point.

Sunday, July 17

"One day at a time." That famous saying is true. One just has to keep on keepin' on. Getting up in the morning is the first big step—that first walk to the bathroom is the worst. But, you have to keep doing daily things to stay ahead. Cooking and laundry and sewing and cleaning and paying bills, and cutting out coupons and doing shopping.

What I noticed from the beginning, I never stopped disciplining my children. Even when I was too sick to stand or raise my head, I was still yelling about dirty socks on the floor. Neither did I lose contact with my friends. I always wanted to know what was happening.

Disciplining in daily exercise is ultra important. When I was too sick to walk, or even stand, I would sort of throw myself on a big mat, and do my exercises with leg weights and dumbbells. Sometimes, I would have to take a nap between the arm and leg exercises. I often think what my Mom had to go through watching her daughter flop around, and struggle even to do the simplest activities.

I got up to 20 minutes on the rowing machine, keeping a timer within reach. Each day when I rowed at the same time, I tested my eyes. A school bus made a stop at the corner the same time every day. Cars passed by. I looked down at my feet and around the room. Every day I noticed the tiniest (I mean tiny!) improvement. The double vision became less double, and then the blurry became less blurry. That is how it has always been. Now, when I get impatient, my mother says. "At least, you are going in the right direction."

I would often do exercises on the rug in my bedroom, right before I went to bed. Many of my stuffed animals were in a group, lined up against the wall, and I imagined them cheering me on and giving me encouragement. Sometimes I talked to my two teddy bears. One only listened, but the other one communicated more. It had one of those give-and-take faces.

For some time now, I've been sleeping with my weights, so I can do exercises first thing in the morning before I get out of bed. I snap on the radio and away I go! It is not easy, but I do it religiously, because I know that this ritual is what makes me strong.

Monday, July 18

I am going to see Dr. Cantu, my brain surgeon to say hello and thanks. He operated on August 26, 1987, and I haven't seen him since September.

Tuesday, July 19

PT. Worked a lot on the Biodex machine. Called California. Linda, my sister, who has Multiple Sclerosis, has to have a hysterectomy. We talked about her condition. I talked her into getting a cane.

Wednesday, July 20

I walked to CVS Pharmacy by myself. Before I left, David said, "Be careful when you cross the streets!" Role reversal. Pretty good. My case for PT extension comes up with Harvard Community Health Plan appeals. I'm not worried. Everything seems to go my way.

Thursday, July 21

Last day at OT. My therapist, Pat White, said I do better than 90% of the patients who come in there, but she doesn't know if I will get back all the way to "normal" again. I told her that I KNEW that I WOULD! Have to take David to see his pediatrician, Dr. Tripp, to check out a lump. He's nervous, and envisions himself with cancer and under the knife. Everything is OK.

Friday, July 22

PT. Getting better on the ankle board. Walked two miles. Started special eye exercises. I'd give anything to get rid of the blurriness and dizziness. I'm refocusing constantly. Appeals case came up today, not Wednesday. David got his palate extender on his upper jaw. He's having a hard time talking and eating.

Saturday, July 23

David threw different sized balls to me in the garage. I used a bat and a tennis racket. We started with a beach ball, and worked down to a tennis ball. I said, "If I can't hit this beach ball, we're really in trouble!"

Sunday, July 24

Played miniature golf with Aubrey, David, and his friend, Don. Got a hole-in-one on the first hole! My difficulty was not in putting, but in walking around. At home, Don, David's friend, gave me some tips on how to go down steps.

Monday, July 25

Today I saw Dr. V. He always makes me feel good. He checked my eyes and said I was better. I gave him a printout of this journal, so far. I always have so much to say when I see him.

Tuesday, July 26

Today marks eleven months since my brain surgery. PT. Doing even better on the ankle board. David practiced more with me in the garage. Batting and tennis, and I was even moving around a little. Did therapy at neighborhood pool.

Wednesday, July 27

HCHP benefit extension approved. No surprise to me. I felt that would be the decision all along. Happy about that! Pool therapy. Tutoring tonight. After Jeffrey and I finished, we played tennis in the garage.

Thursday, July 28

Septic system gets cleaned. I'm proud of myself because I remembered where the location of the entrance was. Last week when I started digging to find it, I hit it right on the button! Then I called David to help dig further.

Friday, July 29

PT. My last day with Jane. I gave her a gold puff heart charm. I am so lucky to have had her. Her expertise, sensitivity and awareness of my needs were unsurpassed. She had a critical eye, and knew just what to do. How do you give constructive criticism to someone who is already suffering from loss of control and loss of self-esteem? Jane did it and she did it with grace and a great sense of humor. The Acton-Boxborough Jamboree started tonight. I saw a hot air balloon as I was coming back from the pool. I jumped rope eight times.

18.

OBJECT OF ATTENTION

Saturday, July 30

The kids went to the Digital Senior Classics (golf tournament) to benefit Emerson Hospital. They saw some old "greats," Arnold Palmer and Chi Chi Rodriguez. Peter said, "Arnold Palmer talked to me." I said, "What did he say?" Peter said that as Palmer was putting close to the ropes, he said, "Could you move a little, son?"

I walked to the A-B Jamboree alone. I mostly visited the crafts area. On the way back home, a woman in a straw hat came up to me, and said, "Are you all right?" I have known her for several years, but I only run into her about every two years. So, she did not know about my past year. She said, "Everyone is staring because you're weaving." I really felt badly.

We sat under a tree and talked for a while, and a thought occurred to me. If people were, in fact, staring, they probably wouldn't have been staring quite so hard, if I were in a wheelchair or had a cane. But, the fact that I was staggering a little, may have given people the notion that I was drunk, or something was wrong. Or, perhaps the heat was getting to me.

It's safe in my neighborhood. It's safe at the pool. It's safe with my doctors and therapists. It's safe with people who are happy just to see me on my feet. But, when you venture to the outside world with "normal" people, then you really do lose your confidence. You are slower. You don't step lively. People live fast, and they are impatient. There is no way that they can really know or understand how it feels.

Michael, David's friend, is here. Both he and David have braces. At dinner tonight, Peter referred to them as the "brace brothers."

19.

HAPPY ANNIVERSARY—
IT'S BEEN A TOUGH YEAR

Sunday, July 31

The kids and their father and Michael leave for Martha's Vineyard. Breakfast with my friend, Judy. Dinner at Aubrey's. My friend, Fran Harris, who lives in his neighborhood, came also. He had marinated shrimp, shish-ka-bob and garlic and parsley pasta. Never enough garlic for me. I walked to his house. 1.5 miles. Thought it was further.

Monday, August 1

It's August! Going to Rockport Shoe Factory in Marlboro with Nancy and Anita. Bought some great shoes. $65 down to $29. Some of us have all the luck.

Tuesday, August 2

Today my sister, Linda, had her operation. Called Mom, and thank God, all is well.

Wednesday, August 3

PT. Only one more time after this to go. I practiced a lot on the steps. Heard from Club Med. The district manager will be contacting me in a few weeks about my ideas. Two suggestions were villages for senior citizens and handicapped people. Can't believe they're still interested after over a year. In April 1987, I sent them a letter expressing interest in promoting Club Med sales. In July the V.P. called. At that time I was very sick with what we thought was Multiple Sclerosis. I will never forget what he said: "Please call back when you're feeling better. We need some aggressively-minded people like you."

Thursday, August 4

Pool therapy.

Friday, August 5

Went out for breakfast with a friend. Kids came back from vacation all tanned.

Saturday, August 6

Today I finally went to pick up my new car. Another Mazda. Both Aubrey and Donna went with me, so Aubrey could drive my new car back. It's blue inside and out, pinstripe, sunroof. Very nice. We stopped to get some gas. People were even gathering around and admiring the car.

Then we headed for the high school parking lot. I drove around feeling excited and a little anxious. What could go wrong in a parking lot, right? Wrong! At a couple miles an hour or less, I was headed for a parking space in front of the wire mesh-type baseball fence. I wanted to stop the car, but I couldn't find the brake. My right foot kept going in between the gas and brake pedals. (I think this is called proprioception.) Before you know it, I was panicking and pumping air.

I crashed into the fence, and I was devastated. When I saw the fence coming towards me, I felt I had no control at all. This was scary. I'm so glad Aubrey was with me. He always seems to know what to do, and he knows how to handle me. Brand new car, minutes old, insurance company, body shop, that is all I could think about.

Luckily, there were only a few scratches on the hood of the car. I am so embarrassed even to be writing this, because I feel so stupid!

We sat in the grass for about an hour. I kept crying as I pulled up blades of grass. I remember telling Aubrey to fix the fence. Being the strong man he is, he bent the fence back into shape. I remember a man from the tennis courts came to us to see if we needed any help.

We got back into the car, and did more practicing. I had to, because if I didn't, it would have been a long time before I would get behind the wheel again. It's always hard to face the risk of possible failure. I waited a few hours before I told the kids. I cried. They said it was "no big deal." Peter jokingly said, "Can I go out and try to *find* the accident?" He came in, and said, "You call *that* an accident?" Probably comparing to his totaling my car six weeks ago!

My confidence was zero before, and now it's -10. I'm surprised by now that I have not clumsily broken something, or fallen down the steps, or hurt myself in another way. Even though *everyone* does something "off" once in awhile, when I do it, I feel it's because of my condition (which it is) and I feel stupid!

Sunday, August 7

Drove the car again. Did much better. Anything is better than yesterday. Feeling a little low. Wonder why?!

Monday, August 8

Aubrey and I took the car back to the dealer. A service man with a white rag hanging out of his back pocket approached us. He said, "Can I help you?" I said, "The scratches on the hood were caused when I rolled into a mesh fence." He said, "I will tell the manager it came off the truck that way". Aubrey knows how honest I am, and he said to me, "Don't say a word!"

Then the man with the tie came out, didn't even look at us, looked at the scratches, and said, "It looks like someone hit a fence. Did you hit a fence?" Aubrey replied, "I didn't hit no fence." I just kept looking straight ahead and down, knowing for sure the manager would see something in my face. It was such a hilarious situation. Anyway, after the service person told us what he was going to tell the manager, we could not say otherwise, as that would be detrimental to him.

Tuesday, August 9

Aubrey goes to the doctor for his hip. He is going to have a hip replacement. I said, "Who is going to take care of you, Aubrey?" He said, "You are!"

Wednesday, August 10

My last therapy session. Going to miss everyone. You get attached. Brought the ankle board home. Pretty soon I am going to have a full-sized gym: rowing machine, mini-trampoline, ankle weights, jump rope, racquet and balls and the neighborhood pool.

Thursday, August 11

Called around. Called Massachusetts Rehabilitation Commission. I think they want to sponsor me for driver's education, and any type of vocational training I may need. Even though I'm busy all the time, I want to work, to be employed. I'm tired of being hauled around, and being so dependent.

Friday, August 12

Finally got my car registration. Aubrey left on vacation to see his family. He'll be back on the 23rd. Went to get ice cream with Judy.

Saturday, August 13

Laundry and housecleaning. Nothing exciting.

Sunday, August 14

My family called. We keep in touch with letters, and talk almost every weekend. My former mother-in-law, Esther, is a real gem, and has kept in touch also. She has been a support and one of my best friends for years. Went shopping with Donna. I always spend money when I am with Donna.

Monday, August 15

Heard from Massachusetts Rehabilitation Commission. Have appointment for interview September 12. Not soon enough, but with vacations and Labor Day, I have to wait. I've noticed I get very impatient with myself. I always want to do things faster. To get them done right now! Maybe this is why I have made so much progress, but people keep telling me, "You're too hard on yourself!" I don't think this is anything new; that's how I've always been.

Tuesday, August 16

Took Boswell to the vet. Pus coming out of his eye and vomiting. Just a little irritation. Nothing serious. Taking Bos to the vet is a family affair; we all go.

Wednesday, August 17

Took David to the doctor for follow-up on ankles. As long as he plays sports, he'll have some problems.

Thursday, August 18

Going for my first haircut in over a year. I ACTUALLY NEED A HAIRCUT! Johanna will do it at her shop. Took my camera. A big event. Before radiation, she came to my house and cut my hair in the kitchen in front of the stove. Though I knew I would be losing my hair in a few weeks, I still wanted to have it cut. She took no money. She said, "Just get better."

Unfortunately, the medication grew hair on my face. My electrologist, Kathy, brought her equipment to my house. She spent hours with me. I probably racked up over $150, but she wanted no money either. A lot less humid. Spent all afternoon at the pool. Not much time in the water. Sun is hot, but air and water cool.

I discovered the source of water leaking in the basement. It was the dehumidifier between the laundry room and the shop located between two walls. I repaired it by aligning the pipe, and shortening up on the wire, from which it hung. Felt pretty proud of myself!

Surprisingly, Bush made a decent speech at the Republican Convention. Think he made a mistake choosing Quayle as his running mate.

Friday, August 19

Took my watch to have the crystal replaced. Makes me mad. Have no idea how I shattered it.

Neighbors gathering down at the pool 8–10 p.m. to socialize. We all sat in a big circle. People brought snacks and drinks. There was music. Twenty people there, but only one went swimming. It was too cold. I wore a sweater.

After I got home I listened to a tape, Paul Simon's *Graceland* and danced in the family room in front of the glass doors, so I could see my reflection. I can SEE I am getting better, and I can feel it.

Improvement happens so slowly, that I know I am going to wake up one day, months from now, or maybe years from now, and say, "When did this all happen? When did I get better?"

Saturday, August 20

Laundry and cleaning.

Sunday, August 21

Spent the afternoon at the pool. Walked 2.7 miles

Monday, August 22

It's getting cooler. 62 degrees. Might reach 70. Wearing a sweatshirt today. Walked 2.8 miles.

Tuesday, August 23

Aubrey's back from vacation. Did pruning in the yard. Sometimes, I have to hold onto the branches to keep my balance.

Peter rode in an 18-wheeler. Moving job. He's had a lot of interesting temporary jobs. He and Joel have a lawn and yard service called Pete and Joel Enterprises. They had a rap on the answering machine with rap music that goes like this: (I think it's cute!)

My name is Joel,
My name is Pete.
When we do a job,
It's done complete.
We don't mess around,
No hassles or surprises
'Cause we are Pete and Joel Enterprises.

Lawn need mowing?
Yard work need done?
We've got the time,
And we think it's fun.

We'll cut your grass,
We'll stack your lumber.
Just leave your name
And your telephone number.

They do a good job, and people like them. They work well as partners. Not really meaning to, of course, but I've heard them talking business with each other, and they sound very professional. I have also heard Peter talking on the phone to his customers. "Sunrise, sunset, quickly go the days."

People are very impressed with David also. David does a variety of services, taking care of pets, lawns and some babysitting. I am always getting comments from everyone about what great kids I have, and how lucky I am. And they are. And I am.

Wednesday, August 24

Spent over two hours with David straightening up his room. and trying on clothes to see if they still fit (mostly pants). Boy, has he grown in the last two months! We're giving away five large bags of clothes. He packs more stuff into that room!

Thursday, August 25

Working on this book all day. It's warming up outside again.

Friday, August 26

Happy Anniversary! Had my brain surgery one year ago today! Made it through one year. Aubrey and I are going out to dinner to celebrate. We're going back to Chez Claude Restaurant. We were there over a year ago with my mom, when I was first diagnosed with Multiple Sclerosis. We'll get a menu and order ahead of time like before, so we don't have to wait. Maybe we'll order rack of lamb like we did last year. We did.

And it was great! The owner, Claude, remembered us, and even where we sat last year. I was so glad that I could have a nice dinner, and not rush out like last time. I remember I was so sick, that we had to go immediately after dinner, leaving Mom's full cup of coffee untouched.

Saturday, August 27

Did a lot of pruning in the yard.

Sunday, August 28

Lynrd Skynrd concert at Great Woods. One of Peter's friends bowed out, so Peter asked David. I always worry when they go any distance.

Monday, August 29

Aubrey took my car to have the scratches fixed. Can't wait 'til I start to drive. Everyone is always kind and asking if I need a ride. However, sometimes I feel like going shopping on the spur of the moment, but I don't have the freedom to do that yet.

Tuesday, August 30

Today I saw Dr. Moore. I still have nystagmus on my right eye and ataxia on the right side of my body, arm and leg. My right eye "shakes (can't focus) when I look to the right, and my right leg "shakes" when I run my right heel down my left shin. Typical neurological tests.

He said the width of my gait is about four inches compared to six inches four months ago. I told him about my accomplishments and frustrations. He said that I made "spectacular recovery" and that I was a "success story." I know I have come a long way, but I have a long way to go. Slow. Slow.

He said I had a lot of determination. He seemed to enjoy the beginnings of my book. I want to be better, and "better" is relative, but I want that total feeling of well-being. Dr. Moore says that it will come, and that the impatience I have is not a bad thing.

A frozen foods salesman came to the house to give a presentation. As I sat down he said, "Bad back?" To which I replied, "No, brain cancer." May just as well have a little fun!

Wednesday, August 31

Groceries. Everyone is always so kind to me, making sure I have rides. Always making sure I don't need anything. Walked 1.5 miles with Patti and her mentally challenged adult daughter, Barbara Jean, who is in a wheelchair. I like kidding with B.J. When walking, I sometimes tend to wander out into the middle of the street. She says in her slurred voice, "Get over here!" I say "Yes, Mommy!" B.J. likes me because I understand her. Took a bathroom break at my house, and then went out for 1.5 more miles. Hemmed David's pants.

Thursday, September 1

Bank and shopping. David had orientation at the high school. Made scallops with sauce over linguine. The kids really love this. Also made tacos filled with eggplant, onions, mushrooms, garlic, green pepper, hamburger and spices. I really "go to town" when I make tacos!

Walked 3.1 miles. I don't know how I do it. I just put one foot in front of the other, and I breathe regularly. I certainly am no picture of grace! Tonight I danced again in front of the window, watching my reflection. I wish my doctors could see me! I dance better than I can walk. I think I can dance better than I can do almost anything.

Friday, September 2

House chores. Emerson Hospital Auxiliary invites me to their luncheon, which will be held September 27. They want me to speak, which I am going to love, because it will give me an opportunity to thank everyone for their meals and kind support to me and my children.

Spent most of the afternoon at the pool. Not many of these days left. Treated Aubrey to soft-serve ice cream. He had a bad day.

Saturday, September 3

The kids drove to Connecticut to see their father. I'm waiting for a call…They just called. They call their father before they leave here, and they call me when they get there. They do the opposite when they come home. I feel better when the bases are covered.

Aubrey and I danced to Paul Simon's *Graceland*. He was truly amazed, and said if I could dance like that, I could do anything. I like the song, "Diamonds on the Soles of her Shoes." That's how I feel when I'm dancing—like I have diamonds on the soles of my shoes.

Sunday, September 4

Kids are back. They did a great job. Rainy and cool. Lower 70's. Can't believe summer is almost over. Talked to my family, some yesterday, some today. Going to make reservations for around Christmastime. California, here I come!

Monday, September 5

Labor Day. Peter can't change the oil in his car, because the stores are closed, so he can't buy the oil. David has organized a bunch of kids to play softball at the high school. Good day for it. He's such an organizer. He just makes tons of phone calls and gets everyone going.

Walked 3.5 miles. I examine every step I take. Where is my foot placement when I stagger? Do I thrust my hip forward enough? Am I walking in the center of my foot? Am I casually swinging my upper torso and my arms? Loose. Loose.

Tuesday, September 6

To the hospital for a CAT Scan. I hate it. I hate going to the hospital. Checking in. Having the IV put in. They have to do this, so the dye can circulate, making the X-rays accurate. The only good thing is the pleasantness of the young women who staff the CAT Scan room. They remember me from the last time, and tell me how well I am doing. As I climb up on the table, I always say, "I forgot how much fun this used to be!"

20.

SCHOOL BEGINS, LIFE GOES ON

Wednesday, September 7

First day of school. David is a freshman; Peter, a senior. First time in years they are in the same school. I got kind of teary seeing David walk off toward the woods to go to school. Yesterday he tried on his clothes for the first day of school, and I took a picture. When I told Peter, he said, "I wasn't that way, was I?" "No." "Oh, good!" When David left for school, Peter was still in the shower. Somehow I can tell what kind of year this is going to be!

Dr. V. called. CAT Scan is good.

The director from Theatre III called. She said, "I have an off-the-wall question for you. Do you want to be in the fall show?" I said, "Sure, if they have a crane to get me on and off the stage." Someone asked the director, "Do you think Diane has the stamina?" To which she replied, "Diane can probably out-stamina all of us!" I was thrilled! This made my day. Maybe next time. As I've mentioned before, I always appear better than I am. Especially if I am just standing and not moving.

Thursday, September 8

David is practicing for the freshman soccer team. He came home with a sore ankle and a few bruises. Did chores. Always seems to be a lot of paperwork. Walked 3.1 miles. Planning to help Aubrey do his résumé. He thinks I should go into the business. I certainly have had a lot of practice doing my own.

Friday, September 9

A neighbor died today. He was getting ready to take a shower, and had a massive heart attack. Left a wife, five children and his mother, who lived with them. No matter how many times there is an unexpected death, people are still continually surprised when it happens. A real shock for the family, friends, and community. His wife sent someone to me to make sure I was OK with receiving the news. In all her grief, she was thinking about me.

Saturday, September 10

Nice day. Did some shopping. Played "Trivial Pursuit" with David. I always call him a "cheater" and he calls me a "cheater."

Sunday, September 11

Today's the wake. Long line. Tons of people. Wonderful man. Another test of this community's strength. The support was overwhelming!

Monday, September 12

Big day. The funeral. Also Massachusetts Rehabilitation Commission. Going to take the time to get all medical reports in to them. Maybe by December or January I can have a driver evaluation test. It's like I have nothing else to do until then! Right! Visit at Fran's. Drugs and alcohol meeting at the school. Pulled David's tooth out with my left hand.

Tuesday, September 13

Massachusetts General Hospital. Dr. Gibai (under Dr. Hochberg) checked reflexes, eyes, and had me do my traditional walk around the examination table. Gave me some brain teasers: "What is 7 from 100?" "93." "7 from 93?" "86." "7 from 86?" He kept going. I wondered how patients would respond if math was not a favorite subject in school. And also whether this test has any validity.

"Spell your last name." "J-E-P-S-E-N." "Spell your last name backwards."

"N-E-S-P-E-J." "Do you want me to spell your name backwards?" "I-A-B-I-G." "What is your area code?" "I always get area code and zip code mixed up, but it's 508." He said in some cases such as mine, that encephalitis develops in the brain. Not so with me.

Then Drs. Hochberg and Smith came into the room. They said that the CAT Scan looked so good, that there was no trace that there ever WAS a tumor! They were all impressed that I was writing a book. Dr. Hochberg asked if Alan Alda was going to play his role when my book became a movie. He looks a lot like him, except probably Dr. Hochberg is more handsome.

Dr. Hochberg wanted me to take the MRI test again, this time with a dye called Gadolinium. My favorite test! Right! I love being rolled into a tube with loud banging noises like a jackhammer. Or visualize yourself being in the trunk of a car, and someone banging on it for an hour! You can imagine how thrilled I was! I said, "I will pay you not to have me take this test." They also wanted me to have a Lumbar Puncture. This is where they draw the fluid out of the spine, searching for cancer cells. Very painful and uncomfortable test. Very bad headaches for days after. One time headaches lasted a month! I absolutely refused to take this test again!

The doctors were amazed at my progress, and said they knew very little about my disease. I said, "Am I doing this for science, taking the tests?" I guess they want to make sure everything is OK. They said, "We don't want you calling us in six months saying you are sick." Also, went to Massachusetts Eye and Ear for an examination.

Wednesday, September 14

Peter has study hall the last period, and wanted me to write a "dismissal note for an appointment." Which I did. He had a lot of things to do, and I thought it was OK, just this once. The vice-principal called me. I guess he became suspicious, because Peter handed the note in late, and because of my feeble handwriting on a piece of math paper.

Thursday, September 15

Peter's first visit to the oral surgeon. Needs to have his wisdom teeth out. Voted in the Massachusetts primary elections.

Friday, September 16

Peter went to Brown University with his friend, Matt LeBaron. They went on a tour and then saw the Brown-Yale soccer game. And back at the ranch, I went to David's soccer game against Concord Academy, a private school. Acton-Boxborough won 7-0.

Had a weird dream (seem to have a lot). When I was dreaming, my "dream memory disk" became full. In order to finish my dream, I had to get another disk, which I did. The floating feeling of actually getting another disk during my dream to finish my dream was incredible! Confusing?

Saturday, September 17

Lots of ironing. Red Sox are 4 ½ games ahead.

Sunday September 18

Nice day, but kind of boring. Worked all day on this book, and then went out for ice cream.

Monday, September 19

Had my fifth draft of the book covered and bound. Judy did it at work. Book not done, but looks great! Gave David a full-body massage. He's had a lot of little injuries with soccer.

Tuesday, September 20

Soccer Boosters meeting tonight.

Wednesday, September 21

Have been feeling kind of numbness in my nose and mouth area. Wonder if it's because I am nervous about my upcoming tests, or if something else is wrong. (Later mentioned this to Dr.V. on September 27. He said that because I was slightly hyperventilating, that caused changes in breathing, and in turn, that numbing sensation.)

Walked .7 miles with 2 ½ lb. weights on my ankles. After I take them off, I walk better. Getting bored. Need to start a project and set more goals.

Thursday, September 22

Walked 1.4 miles with weights. Walking better. Created an experimental résumé questionnaire for interviewing people, to help them write their résumés. I really don't know what I'm doing. I miss the pool and the socialization. I need to be with people. I hate to write so much. My arm tightens up. It's also hard for me to write at the bottom of a page. No support for my arm.

Friday, September 23

Cleaning lady back after seven weeks. She spent six weeks in California, and one week recuperating from her vacation.

Saturday, September 24

Feeling frustrated. Need another big project.

Sunday, September 25

Went to Boston with Aubrey and David. The Copley Place. The Charles River. Aubrey said that they charge only $1.00 for sailing lessons. Some rich man provided the sailboats and funding a long time ago.

Stopped in the Old South Congregational Church on Boylston Street, where both Peter and David were baptized. Saw the woman who took care of Peter in the nursery for three years when we lived in Boston. What lead me to the church on that day, at that time, to find Mrs. Louise Mulligan standing there? The last time I saw her was fifteen years ago when she took care of Peter in the nursery school. We also stopped by our old apartment at 240 Commonwealth Avenue, Boston, where we lived before moving to Acton. From the street, I pointed out Peter's bedroom window to David. (David was born two months after we moved to Acton.)

21.

SUCCESS—
SLOW, BUT SURE

Monday, September 26

Had appointment with Dr. V. today. Had HIV test (AIDS). It was negative when they did the test in the hospital last year, and I'm sure it will be negative again. However, subjecting oneself to any test is somewhat risky. I was told the HIV test is usually done in pairs. Dr. V. said I should have it once a year. He said he had to have it every six months because of his contact with patients. It never ends.

He also said that I had to take the other tests recommended by the "Mass General boys" because I am a "rare bird," and they don't know much about Cerebellum Lymphoma. They just want to make sure I am OK. My immune system broke down somewhere, so therefore the searching and researching continues.

Tuesday, September 27

I was a guest at the Emerson Hospital Auxiliary luncheon at Chez Claude Restaurant. A lot of these women so generously provided meals for me and my sons for months. I wanted to thank them publicly. It was a touching moment and a thrill for me. I cried.

Went to David's first soccer game against Concord-Carlisle. A-B won 4-2. Went to Early College Application Workshop at the high school with Peter. It's sta-ar-r-r-ting!

Got myself a temporary job. A portable computer will be delivered to my house. I will be doing data entry for a man who runs a mail order business, selling tea. He advertises in the New Yorker magazine. Made this connection through his wife at the luncheon.

Wednesday, September 28

HIV test negative. Got by another one. Had a re-evaluation at PT. I was skipping and hopping and running much, much better. Need to work on balance more. Good to see Jane again.

Thursday, September 29

Went shopping with Jo Small. Bought a short black wool coat. I have other nice coats, but they are long, and therefore hard to walk in. I have changed, and so must my style of clothes. My business suits and leather pumps are way in the back of the closet. What an excuse to buy a new wardrobe! A-B won soccer game against Lincoln-Sudbury 4-1. Great game. Nice day.

Friday, September 30

Called literary agents.

Saturday, October 1

Another A-B soccer win. This time against Tewksbury. Going to have some trees trimmed.

Sunday, October 2

Peter and David leave around 5 p.m. to stand in the Red Sox ticket line the night before the morning tickets would go on sale. I wondered whether I had done the right thing as a responsible parent, letting David go, but everything turned out well. Two of Peter's friends also went. I asked everyone to watch over David. It rained. They put together a makeshift tent out of four ponchos and an old shower curtain. They got a taste of the life of the homeless. They got home after 12:30 p.m. Monday.

Monday, October 3

The kids returned with their Red Sox tickets and wet and dirty sleeping bags. They were really tired.

While they were gone, I went to the Mass Eye and Ear for a slit lamp examination. Dr. Newman said everything looked great. She said, "Even though you don't feel perfect, you are a success story!" She went to get Dr. Lessell, who while examining me, noticed "eyelid nystagmus." He then called three other doctors in, and they were all marveling. Later, they took a video of my eyes. Aubrey enjoyed the action. He said, "If we see your face on Channel 2, we're suing!"

Tuesday, October 4

Agent wants to look at first few chapters of the book. First class back to yoga tonight. Trying to do things I ordinarily would do. I figure that as long as I continue doing that, that I'll keep getting better. All the doctors are very cautious and say, "I can't say you will totally recover, but judging how well you're doing, you probably will." I always shoot back, "I *know* I will!"

Wednesday, October 5

Yesterday yoga was great! I couldn't believe I was actually there. I was so thankful. I was able to do everything, except once in a while I had to use the table next to me for support during some of the poses that required balance. I was so excited.

Thursday, October 6

The kids went to the Red Sox game tonight. They lost to the Oakland A's 4-3. They got home at 1:45a.m. Got my hair cut the second time since radiation. Real short on the sides. That's how I like it. David's soccer team won another game.

Friday, October 7

David and his friend, Will, who also went to the game, had to miss their first classes at school. They were really exhausted. Peter was only a few minutes late to school. They all had a full day with soccer practice, basketball, Nautilus, etc. They have so much energy, for things they WANT to do, of course.

Saturday, October 8

Went to buy sturdier eyeglass frames. Aubrey helped me decide what looked good. Made an apple pie. Figured out how to make the dough like I used to. Worked on the computer. Laundry and ironing. Even though I seem to do everything slowly, I get it done. I am just glad I am *able* to do it!

Sunday, October 9

Cut out coupons like I do every Sunday. Double coupons add up. The Red Sox got swept—four games straight.

Monday, October 10

No school. Columbus Day. Getting cold outside. Not looking forward to winter. Harder to get around. Walking every day.

Tuesday, October 11

David's soccer team won again, this time against Westford Academy. In the six games they have played, they have scored four goals every time. My new cleaning lady started. She does a good job, and she is a good person. Yoga. I feel strong. It's just my balance, at times. I'm so proud of myself. I'm as flexible, and probably more so, than anyone in the class. All through my illness, I never stopped moving or exercising.

My dad was buried on this date in 1970 (maybe it was the 12th), eighteen years ago. He died in a car accident. I was five months pregnant with Peter at the time. I wonder if he knows about my life today. He always referred to me as "a-wee-yah", meaning "strong" in Arabic.

Wednesday, October 12

Groceries. Every time I go to the supermarket, it takes me a long time, because I stop to talk to so many people I know, and some I don't know. My weekly trip to the supermarket is a good indication that I am getting better. I am able to leave the cart more often to search for items. Also, I'm walking better down the aisles, and changing direction with more ease. I know I'm getting better daily. But, it is difficult to know, because progress is slow. I notice improvement more on a week to week, or month to month basis, or even looking back a few months ago. Been working hard at my little job. I noticed I have to be more aware of what I type. I probably would have made the same amount of mistakes a couple years ago. However, I come down hard on myself, and blame it on my having had a tumor.

Thursday, October 13

Boswell was barking through the glass door at an injured bird on the patio. It had a hard time standing, and its beak kept opening and closing. I didn't know what to do, but I did know I didn't want Boswell to get it. I scooped it up in a cloth, put it in a bucket and carried it into the woods past the reach of Boswell's line. It looked like a big robin.

A-B won a soccer game against Concord-Carlisle. Kids have their annual checkup tonight. All is well. Dukakis and Bush square off in their second and final debate. Bush is afraid to agree to more debates.

Friday, October 14

To the mall with my friend, Brenda. Newly renovated with two levels. If I know myself, I won't be able to come home without buying something.

Saturday, October 15

Soccer team beat Tewksbury 2-1. Car wash made $1100. Powder Puff game. Senior girls against the Junior girls. Flag football. Boys are the cheerleaders. At the last minute, Peter decided to participate. He wore my wine-colored skirt with an elastic waistband. He also dug up a multi-colored wig he had bought years ago for Halloween. All the guys wore balloons or balls for "boobs." Since Peter is a gymnast, he did some fancy moves and flips. I was so glad to be there. The boys looked so funny doing their routines, and running down the field with sneakers and hairy legs! It was so cute. The Seniors won 28-8.

Sunday, October 16

Met Judy for breakfast. Peter and Joel leave for Connecticut. Besides seeing Peter's father, they went to the Celtics game and visited a college. Soccer parents social. I feel pretty. I work on the computer with the radio on. I tap my right foot to the beat for exercise. The doctors always ask me to tap my feet, comparing the right with the left.

Monday, October 17

Peter comes home. I'm always glad when he gets here. The school called to check up on him. They do that with all the seniors.

Tuesday, October 18

David's soccer team still undefeated. They beat Lincoln-Sudbury. Am doing super! Yoga. Doing more balancing. I feel strong.

Wednesday, October 19

Baked three apple pies. One for the Hosmers, the neighbors across the street. Dick takes our trash to the dump every Saturday. Just kindly and quietly does it. One for Aubrey. And, of course, one for us. Peter said, "I hope the large one in the oven is ours!" I DO make the best apple pies. The secret is mostly in the crust that I learned from my farmer neighbor, Millie Russell, when I just a young girl. It is one of my specialties!

Thursday, October 20

Went to the dentist, then to Acton Medical, and then to the oral surgeon. He said I had a teenage problem. Wisdom tooth is infected. Pericoronitis. That's all I need! Antibiotics and hydrogen peroxide rinse. If things don't clear up by the time I go with Peter to have his wisdom teeth out next week, I have to have mine out, too! Oh, boy! David stayed home from school today. He said he feels "hollow." I think he has a touch of the flu. He was well enough in the afternoon to watch his undefeated team continue their record, but he didn't play. He retrieved the balls and kept the game going. He has such a great attitude!

Back-to-school night. I am so glad I was able to go this year. I told the kids that I could probably only go to two classes each, because I would need extra time in-between to find the classrooms. To my surprise, I was able to keep up with the other parents, climbing steps and everything. I made it to all the periods, and on time. And I don't seem to get tired.

Friday, October 21

No school today. Professional day for teachers. Peter drove to Dartmouth alone—about 2 ¼ hours each way. He liked the school, and he is going to apply. Turns out his tour guide was a good friend of the only person he knows there. Of course, I always get worried when he strikes out on his own like that, but I am a mother. What can I say? I really am so proud of him! He is so independent and he is not afraid to take risks.

Saturday, October 22

Going to dinner with Aubrey at his friend's house. The man is an associate at work. I guess the wife's mother had breast cancer. Great dinner. Great people. Great conversation. It was wonderful.

Sunday, October 23

My friend, John's son, Michael, had his birthday #1. Peter, David and I went for the celebration. We think John is so special, just like family. When Peter and David were nine and six years old, respectively, he stayed with us for three years. His cubicle was across from mine at work. He was twenty years old, and his mother was worried about him driving the long distance back and forth from Fall River. He ended up staying with us, and became a tremendous influence on the lives of my children.

When Peter was driving to the celebration, David took down our entire conversation for a school assignment paper. Even though Peter and I were aware of this, we soon forgot, and just carried on. I mentioned time and again, the cruise control, and a lot of "mother picky" things. I'll bet his teacher enjoyed this one!

Monday, October 24

A-B beat Wayland. Our soccer team is good!

Tuesday, October 25

My yoga night. I'm so strong. The class was divided into partners, and back to back, we had to sort of twine our arms. I found my partner shaking from my strength, so I thought maybe I should let up on her a little. It was a good feeling. Strength is not my problem. Nor flexibility. But balance. Yes, it will come. I'm planning on taking acupuncture again (Did it in the spring of 1987 for what the doctors thought was labyrinthitis. It helped ease some of my symptoms.) Anything to speed things along.

Wednesday, October 26

A-B beat Westford Academy 1–0. This was a toughie. Last game. They're undefeated, and will be getting "champion" sweatshirts and individual team trophies.

Thursday, October 27

Peter gets his wisdom teeth out. All four. Right after, he was "out of it" from the medication and the surgery. He really looked like someone had done a job on him. He was sitting there in a brown stuffed leather chair, looking like a zombie. When we first walked into the office, he had so much life. When I saw him after surgery, it looked as if someone had changed him. Cotton in his mouth. Face swollen. Eyes half closed. Posture slumped a little. Totally motionless. I knew that the doctor did a great job, and that he was still under medication, but I almost cried. I guess I just wasn't prepared for this image. After we went to the pharmacy and got home, he slept for most of the rest of the day. I was tired, too, but, I had to switch the ice from one jaw to the other every twenty minutes. Fill ice trays. Make sure he was comfortable, etc.

I am so glad I was even able to take care of him. The thought crossed my mind about how my mother must have felt seeing me in intensive care with my head bandaged, a skillion tubes coming out of my body, and me just lying there motionless. And she must have been really tired, not only with the strain of her sick daughter, but of running the house, taking care of the kids and the dog, cooking, laundry, giving me my medication, keeping track of appointments, making phone calls, accepting visitors, writing out my checks, going to the hospital, and so many, many other things. I don't know how she did it; how her sustaining energy and sense of humor held out! She was pure strength to me. I love her so.

A couple days ago, I met a woman who had been sick for 3 ½ years. She recently had brain surgery, but the doctors still don't were not able to give her a diagnosis. I asked her if her mother lived nearby, and if she could help. She said, "Yes, she does, but she's too tired."

Friday, October 28

Peter is feeling much better. Worked on his car and his homework. I sewed velcro on his car mat, so that it would stick to the floor and not move around. Championship soccer party tonight.

Monday, October 31

It's Halloween. For me, this means Mass General Hospital. This past Tuesday, my yoga instructor asked if anyone was going to an adult Halloween party. I said, "I am!"

Tonight I had a Magnetic Resonance Imaging (MRI) test, and I dressed up in costume. All black. Pants. Shirt. Hat. Except for a white satin tie-around ghost mask with teeth. I carried a four-foot plastic axe, and wore a button that said, "DRACULA SUCKS." I was really worried about this test, so I had to go in with some control, some confidence. The costume did just that! It drew comments from hospital personnel, patients, and visitors alike. One patient borrowed my axe. He said, "I have to go after that nurse!"

It was not like the time before. I was prepared in every way, including my breathing. It wasn't as bad as the first time in July 1987. Also, at that time I was very nauseated and feared I would vomit as I lie in the "tube," and choke. The test was only about a half hour, and the banging noises didn't seem as loud. After five minutes, they pulled me out to give me an injection of Gadolinium. The doctor said, "What part of the brain did you say the tumor was in, because I can't find anything?" Oh, my God! All right!

Rob, our boarder for a month, arrived from Ohio. He ended up having pizza with the kids, and giving out Halloween candy, while I was at the hospital. He is a good man—sensitive and kind and very giving. One night he went to the high school to play basketball with Peter. Things always seem to go our way. I am going to start writing sporadically, as I am busy with other things.

Wednesday, November 2

Made a pumpkin pie from scratch. From the fresh pumpkin, not the can. I'll never do that again! It was delicious, but too much work!

Friday, November 4

Peter went to Williams College for his first interview. Met his dad halfway. I think he did well, and it was a chance to be together with his father.

Tuesday, November 8

Election day. Bush vs. Dukakis. Bush won. Ran a negative campaign and distorted the issues. People voted their fears.

Went to Mass General for a Lumbar Puncture (LP/spinal tap) Very painful. You have to remain still in a fetal, curled position during this procedure. It is mandatory that you lie flat for a few hours in the hospital before you go home. This is supposed to prevent a big, fat headache, but I still managed to get excruciating headaches for one week or more. One time it was for a month. It was very painful to raise my head from the pillow, so going to the bathroom was a real trial. In talking to others, they had to lie flat for 24 hours, and they still got headaches for two weeks. Fluid is taken from the spine in order to look for those naughty cancer cells. In all the times I have had an LP, no cancer cells were ever found.

Saturday, November 12

Attended a Theatre III performance, *A Funny Thing Happened on the Way to the Forum*. It was the best comedy ever, and I got to see a lot of my friends in the cast after the show. But, the greatest thing was, I noticed my eyes had improved! When I went to the spring show in May, when Mom was here, it was very difficult to watch the show. I had a hard time focusing. Now, it's not perfect by a long shot, but I was thrilled! Now I am ready to take on a movie. It has to be a good-sized theater, and my seat cannot be close to the screen. I think I am ready to give it a try.

Monday, November 14

Met with my Massachusetts Rehabilitation counselor. I will be having an extensive, all day evaluation driving test at Braintree Hospital, in a few weeks to determine if I'm ready to drive. I imagine they will check reflexes and the whole bit. Then, if I am ready, I will take lessons to regain my confidence and practice my driving skills. Can't wait. Driving will give me a lot of independence, and open a lot of doors. However, this is not something I want to rush into. After all I have been through, I don't want to hurt myself or someone else. If it means waiting a little longer, I will.

Nice day. Went for a long walk. People are always out on a nice day, so I always end up doing a lot of socializing. That is what is bad about winter. People hibernate more. Sometimes, there will be an occasional wave in the middle of shoveling a driveway. I am already looking forward to spring and it is not even winter yet.

Tuesday, November 15

I enjoyed raking leaves—2½ to 3 hours. I am *able* to do it, so I enjoy it. No headache today. Hope that's the end. Cramps my style!

Thursday, November 24

It's Thanksgiving! And a lot to be thankful for! Peter and David drove to their Dad's house for their traditional dinner at his club. They like to go to this uppity place, because the waiters call them "sir." Aubrey's kids went to a friend's house with their mother. So, Aubrey brought over some steak, and I made some pumpkin pie with walnut trimming. I suggested we try a movie. I had not been to a movie in 1 ½ years. I thought if we could sit in the back of a big theater, my eyes might be able to focus OK. We decided to go to a movie in Lexington. It was a double theater, and our movie "1969" was upstairs. Were we ever shocked when we got up there! It was the smallest theater I have ever seen in all my life! Five rows deep, five across on each side, and ten across in the middle. We did just fine. Not perfect. But, I was thrilled! I was finally able see a movie!

Sunday, November 27

Peter has an interview with Brown University alumnus in Acton. One question asked of him was, "Why do you think you're so unique?"

Monday, November 28

Basketball tryouts start today for both kids. I have a little cold.

Wednesday, November 30

I get my third haircut since radiation. David's soccer banquet. His team was undefeated, so, he'll get a big trophy.

Thursday, December 1

Acupuncture today. Aggy said I was much better this year than last year. She said she thought that even though the treatments wouldn't make me better tomorrow, they would help speed my progress. I'm for anything that has the remote possibility of helping me.

Friday, December 2

David went to the Freshman Class Dance. I was kidding him, saying, "So, how many girls did you dance with tonight? I want to know!" I like to get him all flustered.

Saturday, December 3

Aubrey and I went to a new Chinese restaurant, and then to the National Honor Society Fashion Show. It was fun. It was a big day.

Sunday, December 4

12:30 p.m. Aubrey and I go to his boss's Christmas party.
4 p.m. Aubrey checks into Emerson Hospital to go under the knife.

Monday, December 5

8 a.m. Aubrey had hip replacement surgery. His arthritis was really bad, and then the cartilage had worn away. He was in a lot of pain and limped, and so was very much looking forward to his surgery. I sent him a card, and wrote, "New Hip, No Skip."

Tuesday, December 6

Saw my neurologist, Dr. Moore. Every time I see him (It's been every three months), I feel that he is so happy for me, that he's jumping out of his skin. Not everyone sees this, because he doesn't appear to be the type. But I can see it, and I can feel it.

I was somewhat able to walk heel-to-toe which I have never done before, and I don't really know if I can do it again! My eyes are far from perfect, but they are getting better. There is less and less nystagmus (involuntary eye muscle movement). I'm just getting better. I know it. It's a nice feeling to leave the doctors' offices, and see their excitement, feel their encouragement, and realize they know and verbalize what I already know, in the deepest part of my soul.

Aubrey looks good. Sore. Had to be transferred to Lahey Clinic to radiate his new hip. Sort of cauterize it. I made him some spinach pizza. I saw it in the supermarket (three small round pieces for $2.29), and read the ingredients: feta cheese, onion and spinach. I decided to make it myself, and it turned out yummy!

Dr. Vaillant, my primary care doctor, and the medical director of Emerson Hospital spoke at Emerson Hospital on "Living Longer and Liking it Better". I was there to hear him because (nominated by him over a year ago) I am a corporator there. He's so knowledgeable and such a good speaker. Everybody loves him. Everybody! After the presentation, I went to shake his hand, but instead, he hugged me. He always does that, and I love it!

Wednesday, December 6

When I was walking up the steps that lead to the second floor at Acton Medical, an old man called to me, as I was about one-fourth of the way up. He said, "Can I help you?" I said, "No thank you," but appreciated his offer. I also felt that it made him feel good that he was able to help someone. On the other hand, I felt that some day, I would like to get past the point of being an object of attention.

Thursday, December 7

Acupuncture. Out to lunch with John, Karl and Dave (engineers I used to work with at Gen Rad). Sort of a belated birthday celebration.

22.

THE BEGINNING OF INDEPENDENCE

Friday, December 9

Some kid fell on David's ankle during basketball practice. We thought that it might be broken. Had to find a ride to Emerson Hospital at 9 p.m. Times like this, I wish even more I was able to drive. No broken ankle. Just a bad sprain.

Wednesday, December 14

Driver evaluation test at Braintree Hospital. Lasted all day. Included assessment of: physical status, reaction time testing, vision, visual perception skills, thinking, reasoning and judgment. I passed! I was recommended for 10 hours of lessons, focusing on especially two areas: gas/brake reaction (as I expected) and use of mirrors. Eye/saccades a little slow. Average gas/brake reaction time is 37/100 seconds; mine was 48/100 seconds. My friend, Donna, took a day off from work to take me to this long appointment. I am so thrilled I will be driving soon! The beginning of independence. Next, a job. A new life.

Went to Peter's basketball game against Xaverian. (How did I have the energy?) A-B won. I can't believe how much stamina I have!

Thursday, December 22

Peter, David, and I fly to California to see my family. What a glorious time! I can't believe I got on the plane without tripping or running into someone. Another first. It felt great! Any time I do something for the first time, I step back, and look at myself, and I can't believe it! Really was quite easy. I guess I was also worried about spilling something on my tray. The real biggie was deciding whether to go to the lavatory, which would, of course, involve walking down the aisle. I did it without any problem, and I was proud.

I loved seeing my mom. It had been since May. I loved spending time with her, doing everything, talking and shopping, cooking and baking, doing exercises and yoga on the floor. I can't believe at over 73 years, she was able to do so much. Lie on your back. Swing your legs straight back over your head, and touch your toes to the floor. Well, she can do that! Incredible! I couldn't believe it! I had to take a photo.

Since Georgia, my younger sister, and her family were all sick, they couldn't join the rest of us for Christmas. Rising to the occasion, I hopped the plane to go to them. I couldn't believe I was flying all over California! At the small airport, I had to deplane using steps, instead of walking off onto a ramp as one usually does. I felt like President Reagan! For those two weeks, it was mostly cold and rainy in California, but as for me, I was with my family, and the sun was shining.

Thursday, January 19, 1989

Big step today. I renewed my license. Now I am ready to go out with an instructor from the hospital. Ten hours of training recommended. I can't believe I am doing this! Except for about a couple of months somewhere in-between, it's been about two years for me. I'm scared. I'm headin' for the highways. I have already warned my friends!

It's hard to know where to stop with this book. People marvel at my progress, and ask me how I do it. I don't feel as if I am doing anything extra special. From the beginning, even when things seemed impossible, and I wanted to die, somehow the next day came. And there were things to do. Simple things, like eating meals, going to the bathroom, exercising, deciding what side to lie on, chewing gum to try to exercise my jaw that was slightly numb and tingly. Then, it was trying to make it to the next mailbox with my walker, then a four-pronged cane, and finally a regular cane. Then walking around the block. Talking to people, opening cards, paying bills, keeping appointments, all kinds of doctors, treatments, therapy, tests. My kids' schedules—school, sports, banquets, their friends.

School starts. Leaves fall. The driveway needs plowed. Christmas comes and goes. Spring is here. Then summer. I get out and walk more. And then the whole thing starts all over again.

I guess I just couldn't fit dying into my schedule! There is too much living and loving to do. I find that now, more than ever. I take the time to listen more carefully, even to a stranger in the supermarket. I really appreciate the little things I am able to do, like showering without a chair, and cooking my own meals. But, knowing me, I won't be satisfied until I can kick my foot over my head! I like being able to stay up late, so I can catch up on some "gab" time with the kids.

I feel a tiny bit better every day. Things go my way. I know "the sun'll come out tomorrow." And I know this gift of life is not without a purpose. I believe I will be used as an instrument of faith to give others hope, so that they may have the courage and the strength to take control where they can.

23.

ONE MOMENT IN TIME

Friday, February 10

The date has been set for the beginning of my driver's training, March 7, I'm kind of scared. It's been a while. David already has me "reserved" to take him to the athletic club!

Went to two basketball games today. David's team lost in overtime on the last second. That was a heartbreaker! He played great, though, and put in two three-pointers. Peter's team won, but not as big as some of the games where A-B scored 101 and also 104. At the first game, Peter put in the basket that took the team to 100 points. The crowd was going mad, yelling and stamping their feet, when the score was tied at 99. What happened was, one A-B player missed the shot, and then Peter put in the rebound. The second game was 104-79 in Bedford. This game was so exciting with A-B scoring 15 three-pointers, and Bedford scoring about six.

Peter got to start in the Wayland game (and played a good part of it), because the coach was unhappy with the usual starting players. They would always be tardy, and Peter was always early. He did a great job! It was his game! David starts with the junior varsity every game, and also does a fabulous job! He's the shortest player on the team, but I think he is the best! No bias here! He hit a couple critical foul shots at the end of the Lincoln-Sudbury game, and assured A-B of a win.

Yesterday during practice, Peter got a cut over his eye, right under his eyebrow, and had to have three stitches. After looking in the mirror, he said, "I wish it were down a little." I said, "Why?" After which he replied, "So it would be more noticeable." How funny is that?!!

Tuesday I went to Mass General for a check-up, and wowed them again! First time without having to take in a recent CAT Scan. My traditional walk around the examining table was much improved from a few months ago. My neurological tests, including eyes, hands and feet, were also noticeably better. The results from my LP (lumbar puncture), sometimes known as spinal tap, were very good, not even showing a trace of protein. I don't really understand what that means, but I know it is wonderful and amazing!

I had been reading where it is good for doctors to become more compassionate toward patients. They are even teaching them in medical schools that this helps healing, especially in cancer patients, and that compassion has a place in the mechanics of medicine. I suppose I should apologize to my doctor, Dr. Gibai, because I shook him up when I asked him for a hug. He seemed very uncomfortable, so I made light of it. I said I had read that hugs were good for cancer patients, but since I was not sick anymore, he did not have to hug me. (In retrospect, instead of asking him for a hug, I should have asked him if he ever hugged his patients. That way, I wouldn't have put him on the spot. But, I didn't think quickly enough.) He then said, "It's a personality problem." I said reassuringly, "Well, you can WORK on that!" He said, "Yes, I think I can." It was the funniest thing. As I laughed, walking down the hall, I thought that maybe I was too loud. It somehow seemed out of place laughing in a place where there was so much pain.

Before I left the room, Dr. Hochberg came in at the end of my appointment. He said, "It is such a pleasure having you as a patient." I said, "It's my pleasure, too!" He told me that I had to have an MRI test (my favorite!) two weeks before my next examination. MRI scheduled for May 26. Appointment June 13. And then thereafter, every eight months just to make sure everything is OK. So, I'd better set my mind accordingly. I guess I should be pretty used to this by now. As he left, I said, "Where is your white coat?" (He had on a suit and tie. I have never seen him without his white coat.) He just turned to his partner and grinned, and walked out. I suppose I should be a little easier on them, but it's fun, and I feel strong, so why not?

My mentally challenged friend in my neighborhood, whom I have mentioned, found out recently that she had to have surgery. (We didn't know at that time that she had breast cancer.) I said, "How do you feel about that?" She said, "Sad." I said, "I would feel sad, too, but you can think some good thoughts." She said, "Where do I get them?" I said, "From within yourself, and I will send you some."

Minuteman Ridge annual pot luck and meeting coming up. They said, "You don't have to bring anything. I said, "Why not? I probably bake more than anyone else around here." I decided to make Tabouleh (a Middle Eastern salad) using the fine ground wheat that my mother brought me from California in her suitcase months ago.

Basketball banquet. I couldn't go to Peter's last year, and only to the awards part of David's. This year, since they are both in the high school, it will be only one banquet, and I will be there. I'll probably cry like I always do. I'm such a crybaby!

At the games, I tie bells attached to a leather string around my wrists, so that when I clap they make noise. I love to hoot and holler, and I love to sit next to someone who likes to do the same.

It's midnight again. I heard the clothes dryer go off downstairs. It's hard for me to get to bed before midnight. I have good intentions, but I never do. Most of the time, I seem to have a lot of energy. I pay for this in the morning, though. I get up with the kids, and some mornings I get them up, but then I go back to sleep. A couple hours later, I wake up and feel as if half the day is gone. But, I can't seem to get into sync.

I am always aware of my dreams before my second awakening. I have some really weird ones. Maybe I should keep a dream journal. Peter just came home. Maybe that's one reason I stay up. I am sure if the whole family turned in early, I would, too. But, I guess that explanation doesn't hold water because I am up during the week days, too. Oh well, nice try! I don't sleep with my weights anymore. The discipline of it got to be too stressful, so I stopped. Instead, I get my exercises in at varying times throughout the day, incorporating walk, dance, yoga, trampoline, rowing machine and Theraband. And just being aware of every step I take, every move I make. Hey! I think I'll write a song!

My balance is getting better. I am able to climb some steps without a railing. This feels good. Also, especially going down, I really need to concentrate on the placement of my right foot (proprioception). I need to kind of throw it out as I take each step, so I don't rub my heel on the back of the step.

Going from Los Angeles to Sacramento airport, when I was going to visit my brother, Jim, I happened to sit next to Emelio, head of the rock group, Tower of Power, and his wife, Thelma. He had his saxophone case, and I remember she was wearing red leather pants and black high heels. We didn't talk until the end of the short plane trip. When I got to Jim's house, we saw in the paper where Emelio was appearing that night with Huey Lewis. The tickets were $25. They said they also played in the Boston area, and invited me to come and see them sometime. Last week, he was introduced as one of the saxophone players on "The David Letterman Special." The program wasn't too exciting, but seeing him for a few seconds made it worth it! At his introduction, he tilted his head back as he played, as if to acknowledge. I couldn't believe it! I was seeing Emelio on the Letterman show, and not too long ago, I was sitting next to him on the airplane!

I like Whitney Houston's song, "One Moment in Time." I sing it, and get teary, because I identify with it.

"Give me one moment in time,
When I'm all I thought I could be,
When all of my dreams are a heartbeat away,
And the answers are all up to me......"

Sunday, February 12

I just wanted to record a moment that happened tonight at The Minuteman Ridge Homeowners Association, my neighborhood's annual meeting and pot luck. I had the opportunity to thank about 100 fellow residents for their food and support and prayers. Of course, being the sort of person I am, I got very teary. Then, after a few seconds of silence, all of a sudden, my emotion was followed by a burst of applause. Everyone was standing. I will never forget that moment as long as I live—friends and supporters cheering! I was cheering them for their support, and they were cheering me. What a feeling!

I was telling Aubrey that even though this has been the worst year of my life, it actually has been the best, also. It's a real different feeling. Almost spiritual. I seem to be more aware of everything, more in tune, more complete. I have even more of a sense of humor than I had before.

I am stronger now, more confident of myself (except when I think of starting to drive again!) I feel I have a special purpose in life, and this is evident to me every day,

Everyone wants a copy of this book for themselves, and then to pass on to someone else. I am still working on getting it published. Since I am not a former author, famous person or movie star, this may be difficult. I may have to set up a press in my garage!

24.

FIRST ATTEMPTS

Tuesday, February 14

Valentine's Day. One of my favorite holidays. David had a basketball game today. After the game, he gave me a wait-a-minute gesture. He went down to the locker room, and brought me back a single white carnation. Later, at home, Peter said, "Where did you get that carnation?" David said, "From a girl at school." Peter said, "How much did you pay?" David rolled his eyes, and said, "You wouldn't want to know." Peter asked, "A dollar?" I guessed, "Five dollars?" He shook his head "yes". I said, "Oh, David, my heart is broken. I don't want you to feel you have to buy me anything. You could just make me a card." David said, "I was desperate!" I was a little perturbed, as I thought $5 was a pretty hefty price to pay for one carnation, and that the girl took advantage of David's strong desire to give that carnation to me. "So, who is this girl anyway? I want to know." Later, when I was alone with David, I told him that was the nicest thing that anyone had ever done for me. I will never forget my $5 carnation.

Peter made me a card on white lined notebook paper with this poem:

> Here is a card
> From me to you;
> If it's too messy,
> Why don't you sue?

This came from
The bottom of my heart;
When you read this line
Please don't rip it apart.

Well, it's Feb. 14.
What else can I say?
Except for the words
Happy Valentine's Day.

Pretty nice. I am so proud of my kids!

Friday, March 3

My driver's training was canceled. Funds were cut at Braintree Hospital and this particular department was one that was eliminated. Of course, it would happen four days before I would begin. I called Massachusetts Rehabilitation, and found that, not only did they not know about my scheduled lessons, but neither did they approve them. I have an appointment to meet with my counselor on the 13th. Soon it will be approved, maybe within a month I will take training through another organization. In the meantime, I will just keep getting better every day.

Sunday, March 5

This is one of those days I'm feeling improvement in my walking. Also, my "spatial" feeling is getting better. Maybe this is an improvement in the vestibular system (learned this term at Mass Eye and Ear), which would, in turn, mean improvement in my balance and my eyesight.

Wednesday, March 8

Boswell, my dog, had surgery today. Had a sebaceous cyst removed from the top of his head. The growth on his cheek was unidentifiable. The vet had to send the sample to Tufts University to have a biopsy taken. Will find out Monday. Poor Bos. He must have known something was up, because his whole body was shaking like mad in the car and at the vet's office.

Thursday, March 9

Had an interview with Emerson Hospital today for part-time employment, but the jobs were just not for me. Either the hours weren't right, or it required a lot of writing, or it took too much coordination, or it wasn't creative enough, or a combination of all of these. I mentioned the idea of a resume writing service, which would incorporate creativity with the use of the computer. The Director of Resources thought it was a good idea. I think I'll work on it.

The basketball banquet. The seniors were especially honored. Peter's coach said even though the season was over, and even though Peter probably would never play college basketball, Peter still was asking how to improve his game. When the principal, Dr. McNulty spoke, he said, "The coach was not going to take more than five or six seniors. Peter said, 'No way, not me!' (meaning he was not about to be left out.). He worked and hustled, and the coach had to go back on his word for the very first time. Now, that's character!" The seniors received pictures of the team in a walnut frame, jackets in school colors with leather sleeves, specially designed watches and certificates.

Description of the watch: Picture the face with numbers on it, but instead of numbers there were abbreviations of their opponents, with A-B in bolder letters at the twelve o'clock position. In the center was an outline of the state of Massachusetts, and a sketch of a basketball entering the net. Really classy!

David got a trophy for "Unsung Hero" for the freshmen team. His coach said a lot of complimentary things about him, and then said, "I wish I knew about those three-pointers earlier!" David became good at shooting from a distance, because of his height. At one time, he was the shortest on the team, and so always got elbowed and banged up under the basket. This led David to shoot further away from the basket. His pediatrician told me that he would grow eight inches in one year!

Friday, March 10

Walked 3.5 miles today. Weather is getting nicer. Ah, spring!

Saturday, March 12

Today I discovered that Dr. Bernie Siegel was coming to Boston to promote his new book, "Peace, Love, and Healing." His seminar is sold out. Maybe next time.

Wednesday, March 22

A couple days ago, I was feeling sorry for myself, because of my limitations, and because I am not like I used to be. Then, in the wee hours of the morning, I wrote down the things that I have done in the last year:

o   Wrote a book.
o   Bought a car.
o   Sold a car.
o   Bought another car.
o   Took driver's training.
o   Flew all over the state of California.
o   Worked at home, part-time job for a few months.
o   Learned to walk again.
o   Gave two speeches.
o   Got rid of my bifocals.
o   Interviewed for a job.
o   Started a resume writing business.
o   Attended plays, seminars, parties.
o   Had physical and occupational therapies.
o   Made new friends—young and old.
o   Bought a painting.
o   Shoveled the driveway.
o   Raked the lawn.
o   Visited people in the hospital.
o   Attended yoga classes.
o   Bought an adult trike.
o   Did aqua-exercises at the pool.
o   Walked 3.6 miles
o   Lived through son's college applications.
o   Nursed my son through extraction of wisdom teeth.
o   Nursed my dog through removal of a tumor.
o   Baked more than I ever have.
o   Continued to raise two teenage boys as a single parent.

I guess I haven't done too badly!

Friday, March 31

Received a reply from a letter I sent to Bernie Siegel. With a purple magic marker, in large letters, he wrote, "Your doctor helped save your life by telling you to keep a journal." He then wrote the name and address of his agent and publisher in New York. He signed it, "Love, Bernie." I framed it, and also copied and framed it for Dr. Vaillant. He was so appreciative of those words from a famous author and renowned doctor.

David is having an impromptu party tonight. He prefers to call it a "get-together."

Monday, May 2

Today I registered my résumé writing business as "Impressions" with the state of Massachusetts, at the Acton Town Hall. I never made any money, because I did it for free a lot of the time.

Friday, May 12

Well, I bought another car, a 1987 Golf GT. It's automatic, black with red trim, sunroof, air conditioning, 4-door, hatchback, 23,000 miles. The dealer is very reputable, and they take care of their people. It is located in Maynard, about three miles away. Three brothers own the business. They are going to build up the gas pedal for me so that it is more even with the brake, as I continue to get better, they will pare it down, if necessary.

My driving instructor quit on the spot. I guess there was a humongous disagreement, but I believe things like this happen sometimes. I heard the director's story, and I heard hers. She really was more qualified to do something other than what she was doing. She wasn't working up to her potential, and my guess is, she wasn't very happy with herself. She is a psychotherapist, and has a very impressive background in social work. After contracting colon cancer three years ago, she halted her private practice, and then temporarily decided to become an instructor. The ironic part is that when I last saw her, she gave me her old résumé just to look at. But, knowing the person I am, the blood started boiling, and the mind started churning. I saw changes I wanted to make right away. I updated her résumé. She was glad because she needed it immediately.

As I sit here typing this, I am in my new office. I bought office furniture: pecan laminate with acrylic-coated ebony surface, office chair, file cabinet. Basically, it is three pieces attached together: a printer table, a corner table and a desk. Add a plant, two lamps, a typewriter on a table, a computer, printer, office supplies, and voila! It's beautiful, functional, and looks so professional. I am so thrilled! I am finally doing something where I feel I am working up to my potential. Also, it is exciting and creative at the same time. What more could I ask for?

Last week I went to an all day seminar on "Right-Brain, Left-Brain." Left-Brain people are more analytical, logical, and usually deal in jobs, such as finance; Right-Brain, more creative, emotional types. In this category, you will find artists, teachers, social workers, and writers. The interesting thing is, the more Right you are, the more you are a night person. Same with motion sickness, which is certainly true for me. The more Right you are, the higher degree of motion sickness. One can be far Right or far Left, or a little or a lot of each. Everyone fills out a questionnaire ahead of time, and the director/instructor does a profile on each person. Aubrey gave me the form, not too many days before my surgery in 1987, but I was unable to attend, of course, at that time. So, they kept calling me periodically.

Many companies schedule their employees to go to these seminars. The individual profiles enable the people to know themselves better. More importantly, they might discover that just because someone else does things differently, or attacks a problem in a different way, that does not mean anyone is wrong.

It normally costs $250 per person, but I was invited free of charge because my profile showed that I was so extreme Right-Brain, and they needed me to contribute to the structure of the group. The instructor needed equal amounts of three groups: Rights, Lefts, and In-betweens. Lecture, videos, a lot of participation, and a fun-filled day!

The seminar was held at Bentley College in Waltham, and since it was right next to Aubrey's work, he gave me a ride. This seminar is presented about once a month, and Aubrey went about a year ago, so we had a lot to talk about.

Peter just got accepted to Bucknell University in Pennsylvania. Now he has to choose between the University of Vermont and Bucknell. His decision should be made within a week.

I've been continuing my yoga classes, and I can see my balance is improving s-l-o-w-l-y. Actually, it is yoga and vigorous exercise for two hours, and it is really a workout!

I still find it difficult to climb steps, especially without railings. It's the placement of the right foot that is not "there" yet. I am getting better though. Sometimes, I will experiment and carry a full basket of clothes up from the basement. Half way up there is a wall on each side, so I feel secure in doing this. No hands on railing, Mom! I have to be careful I don't fall. Going up is easier than going down.

My next MRI test is June 9. Gibai and/or Hochberg, my Mass General boys, on June 13. Driving test on June 22 at 10 a.m. Finally, on May 26, Dr. Bernie Siegel. He has written a couple books on exceptional cancer patients. Oh, yeah, that's me, and will be giving a workshop at Fitchburg State College, a half hour from here.

Finding out what I want to do, and setting up my business and office, has been more exciting than a Club Med vacation. And for me, that's a big step! Just reflecting, I am probably happier and more content with myself and with others, and with the wholeness of life, than I have ever been in my life.

Saturday, May 13

Went to Theatre III to see "Chicago." It was a great show, as usual. They really do professional work there, from directing, casting, costumes, lighting, etc. I have never seen so many multi-talented people in one place. I think of how it was when I was performing, singing and dancing, being a part of a developing script. I know that someday I'll be back. Every time I go to watch a performance, I feel so special because all of my friends come up to me and ask me when I am coming back. There's a tap workshop this summer, and they want me to get some flat tap shoes. They said it would be good for my coordination. Hm-m-m. I don't know. Maybe next year. I seem to be handling a lot of "firsts" in a short period of time.

25.

BACK TO THE BASICS

Monday, May 15

David's been playing baseball. He's really never played on a team before. Not even T-ball. He's enjoying it, and he's the best on the team. No bias here, of course.

Last night Boswell came upstairs and bugged me. He usually doesn't do that, especially lately, now that he is getting older, and has a hard time climbing the steps. Something must have been going on around that time (around 3:30 a.m.) because David got up at the same time. He said that he heard a playground-type ball bouncing outside about 30 times. I asked how he knew it wasn't another type of ball, like a basketball. He said that this ball had more of a "ring" to it. He also saw a flash of light on the walls in his room. He kidded, and said that maybe it was a UFO coming to abduct him. But, the curious thing is that both David and Boswell were reacting to SOMETHING!

Peter chose not to go to the prom this year. He went last year. He said, "Not much bang for the buck!" Some girl asked him to go. He turned her down, and later found she next asked one of his friends. Peter said, "See they don't care who they go with; they just want to go." I tried to explain to him the waiting position women find themselves in, no matter what age. But, I don't think it sank in too well. However, he did go to the beach the next day, with his friend,

Joel, who also chose not to go to the prom. There, they joined other kids, mostly who had partied the night before. He came back red where he missed applying the lotion. The weather was nice, and he had a good time.

Yesterday was also Mother's Day. I always ask for cards, if I don't think they're coming. David made a card with flowers inside, and Peter wrote this in his card:

> Roses are red
> Violets do grow;
> What color is your flower?
> Well, I don't know.
> Today's Mother's Day
> But, it's almost up;
> So, get your nags in,
> And then please shut up.
>
> That was just a joke
> So, don't break into a cry;
> But, if you start up
> Your left brain is the reason why.

Wednesday, May 17

A couple weeks ago I asked Dr. Moore if I would ever ride a bike. He shook his head yes. I asked, "About five years?" He said, "This summer. Just get some training wheels, and put them on a regular bike." "Well, I was thrilled that he thought I could do this, but I don't know if I am ready yet, as I seem to have a lot going on right now.

Thursday, May 18

After having a disaster for a first driving instructor, my second one got fired or quit. I have a third one, and despite everything, all is turning out well. My road test is on June 22.

I seem to be consistently improving, however slowly, on every level, day by day.

It's ironic that Peter was getting his driver's license, just when I was getting sick, and now I am learning to drive again, now that he is off to college. What

I am saying, is there will still be a driver in the house. Amazing how things seem to take care of themselves.

Today was "Stand Up Day" at the school. There was a contest for all the students to design a T-shirt, front and back, showing the dangers of alcohol and drugs. The two winners would receive scholarships, and they would also have their designs on T-shirts. Various companies sponsored this event, and all the kids, staff, and administration of the entire school, each one, was given a shirt to wear today. About 1,200 students. Cost about $9000. Peter said it was an "eyesore!"

Peter and all seniors just have two more days of school. It's 12:30 a.m. and he just went to bed. I can't believe the tests and papers he has right up to the very end. On Monday, May 22, the last day, all the seniors will run down a hill behind the school, and then they go home. This is the way they end the day, and this is the way they end the year. It's tradition. They do it every year. I am not going to miss this one. I saw it one year, and I will tell you what it looks like—a stampede of charging elephants and a lot of dust.

Wednesday, May 24

Peter had to make a decision to go to the University of Vermont, or Bucknell University. In order to attend Bucknell, he had to send back his acceptance, on or before May 24. So, one guess when he made the big D. That's right—today!! Bucknell gets him.

Friday, May 26

Today I attended Dr. Bernie Siegel's workshop. There is too much to discuss here, but I'll just say, there should be more Bernie Siegel(s) in this world. The day was charged with ideas and information and feelings described in his book, *Love, Medicine, and Miracles.* During break, I gave him a copy of this manuscript, got a couple hugs, and took a couple photos. Someone took a picture of him giving me a hug. I noticed he had a huge belt buckle that said "BERNIE." When I shook his hand, I said, "I'm so excited to see you that my heart is pounding!"

Saturday, May 27

The pool opened.

Sunday, May 28

David hurt his right thumb on a grounder during the second inning of his baseball game. This really put him out of commission. He had a problem eating, tying his shoes, doing homework, not to mention he couldn't be involved in sports.

Acton-Boxborough's Baccalaureate was tonight. A senior's speech on "Milestones" was good, and the concert choir and the string quartet were not bad. However, the homily was horrible. There was mention of Lt. Calley and the My Lai Massacre and Oliver North and the Iran-Contra affairs. The main idea or lesson was that the students should mainly listen to their hearts, and just not blindly follow orders. I thought that it was political, and very inappropriate. The best part of the whole night, and I'll never forget this, was being with Peter and sitting next to him, all by myself.

Friday, June 2

Peter's graduation, the Acton-Boxborough class of '89, was scheduled for today at 5:30 p.m. Stormy rains and hurricane-force winds came and dissipated in one hour, and then the sun came out. But not before the 355 seniors were told that graduation exercises were postponed until the next night. Scheduled parties were still attended, and Peter spent the night with about 30 kids with sleeping bags.

Saturday, June 3

A beautiful, gorgeous day! Perfect day for graduation. The boys were in blue caps and gowns on the left, and the girls were in white on the right. I went an hour early, and sat in the third row in the reserved section for the parents. I was so proud. I didn't cry, but I got a little teary during the processional. The feeling I got that was the strongest, was the thrill that I was *able* to be there.

David had gone to the Red Sox baseball game. He barely got back for the beginning of graduation. I told him "If you're late, come as you are." And so he did, in his Red Sox shirt, not feeling awkward or out of place.

More parties, of course.

Sunday, June 4

Today David "umped" his first baseball game. Since he chipped the bone in his thumb, he has been out of commission as far as playing on the team.

However, he was asked to be the plate umpire. His team, the Minutemen, were playing against another Acton team. I felt his decision to do the job took a lot of courage for two reasons. He has never had any experience umpiring, and knew that he would probably be subjected to criticism and confrontation. Secondly, he had to call strikes on his own team members. He did a great job, and made $30 taboot, because the plate umpire didn't show. I was so proud of him for taking on the challenge, coming out on top with confidence in himself, and gaining respect from players and coaches alike.

Mom and Dean moved from their home in Northridge near Los Angles to Ocean Hills Leisure Village near San Diego.

Friday, June 9

Driving lesson. About 1 ½ hours. This counts as a double lesson. I have one more next week; then my road test in Cambridge at 10 a.m., June 22. My instructor says I am doing very well, that I just needed to build up my confidence.

MRI (Magnetic Resonance Imaging) test 6 p.m. at Mass General Hospital. My last MRI was the evening of Halloween, and I dressed in a costume for the occasion. It made me feel powerful and in control. But this time I couldn't think of anything, so I just wore a very comfortable pink cotton outfit. The test was not bad at all. In the beginning, I closed my eyes as they rolled me into the tube. However, this time, I was able to open them, and sort of glance around and observe the inside of the tube.

It really helped when the technician called out how many minutes each segment of the banging (caused by the lining-up of the magnets to take the next picture) would take. There is a microphone in the tube; he can talk to me, and I can talk to him. After this was over, a short 35 minutes this time, I went to Harvard Square and bought a short white skirt and a pair of canvas shoes with ribbons that tied around the ankles. Then I treated Aubrey (He's the one who always treats me.) to dessert. I might as well take advantage of this situation, and buy myself something, and also do something fun every time.

Monday, June 12

This is one way I see my kids: Peter is like a rough and dangerous wave that surfers like to ride. David is like a subtle, foamy wave that gently washes up to the shore.

Tuesday, June 13

Yesterday Peter had a moving job that took him from here to the very northern part of Maine (summer job with a moving company). It was a 7 ½ hour ride. Someone else drove the truck, and they both had to spend the night in Maine. I talked to the woman who handles all the scheduling and office business, and she told me how much they liked Peter, how they always get such a kick out of him, and how he is full of energy. That's always nice to hear. He's handling his lawn service business, too, so he is working seven days a week, unless he is spared by a rainy day. He still finds time for "lifting" at the club, and his friends. Right now he is at the Red Sox game.

He just received freshman registration and course information from Bucknell. Now he just has to find the time to make decisions and fill out forms. I had a talk with him today. I said, "You have been the oldest male in the family for quite some time now, and have held an unspoken position of responsibility, not assumed by a kid in a two-parent home." I told him that when he goes away to school not to worry about me, not that he would, but I wanted to verbally release him of a burden, if it existed. I also talked to David about this. Even though he will naturally be taking on more responsibilities, in his new "role," he shouldn't feel overburdened.

David has recovered from that chipped bone in his thumb, and is now able to play sports, wash his own hair and apply his own deodorant. He became aware of how inconvenient it was to use his left hand for everything, and was also surprised how easily the left hand took over, and became his preferred hand.

Today David has his last full day of school. However, he has exams that end on Monday. He got a good start this year—academically, athletically, and socially.

Today I saw Drs. Gibai and Hochberg at Mass General. Dr. Gibai said, "I have great news! Not only is your MRI good, but it's better than good!"

I said, "So, what does that mean, good and better than good?" He said that my last MRI showed some scar tissue, but in this last one, he could hardly see anything. He was all excited, and sort of jumping with glee, totally out of character! I could not imagine Dr. Gibai with his serious personality doing that. (I think I have changed him a little!). He did other neurological tests, and he was just totally amazed by my progress, including my walking. It was a gloomy day for most people today, but it was not gloomy for me. I know how I feel, and I know I have boundless energy, and I know I am doing well. But, it is always uplifting to get a second opinion, especially if it is a professional one.

Of course, Dr. Gibai had to run out and get Dr. Hochberg, who looked tanned and great, as usual. I said, "Don't you ever work? Every time I see you, you look as if you just got back from a vacation!" Dr. Gibai later told me that Dr. Hochberg was the most disciplined man that he has ever met. Plays tennis three times a week, and takes a one week vacation every two months. I said, "Well, he has to do it, if he has to see people like me all day!"

Anyway, when Dr. Hochberg entered the room, he shook my hand, and said with a little smile on his face, "Well, you can't argue with success." When I am "recovered," I will miss my doctors in many ways. When you think about it, a lot of rapport and respect and communication had built up starting with a sick person who needed help. Then it quickly became more than that.

Sunday, June 18

Saw the movie "Dead Poets Society" starring Robin Williams. Great movie. I didn't even notice any problem with my eyes during the entire movie. I think sitting on the right side of the theater helps, as I favor my left eye.

Tuesday, June 20

Today I take my road test. Today I passed my road test. Except for about a month and a half in the summer of '87, I haven't driven in over 2 ½ years. So, needless to say, I've made a giant step. People don't understand. They say, "It's just like riding a bicycle. You never forget." But, I am not the same person; I am neurologically not the same. Granted, age changes people's reaction time, etc., but that is more a gradual process, and so therefore one compensates, and deals with the change gradually. However, if one has been injured or struck down quickly, this sudden change makes it more difficult to "get back on the bicycle."

I can't believe I'm driving! The poor woman who also went to the registry at the same time I did, failed the test, and was really disappointed. She started to go down a "Do Not Enter" street. That is definitely a no-no. I was a little nervous, but I did better than I ever thought I could. Talking, I think, gives me confidence. I enthusiastically volunteered to be tested first. I need to know the instructor/tester's name to make the situation a little more personal. And when he said, "Do you remember how to do a 3-point turn?" I said, "Of course, I do!" It's always an exciting challenge for me to warm up the cold ones.

My first drive was to the town dump (most residents take their own garbage to the dump), then the post office, then the town hall. There I had to change the name of my résumé-writing business from "Impressions" to "Impressions of Acton." The reason being, when I called the Secretary of State's office to check to see if anyone had that name already, I was informed that the name "Impressions, Inc." was already in use. My fault. Should have called sooner. No problem. Just had to make some phone calls. Yeah! Independence. I love it!

David's baseball team finally lost in the playoffs to Northboro. They did a great job, and were not even expected to go this far. This was the first time David had ever played organized baseball. Not because I'm his mother, but from an unbiased point of view (I'll bet you think I can't do that!), he was definitely the best and most versatile player on the entire team. Fielding and batting and thinking. I'll be on his team any time. The main thing is, he enjoyed playing so much.

Tuesday, July 4

Independence Day. The 4th of July. Today David and his friends went to see the Red Sox baseball game. They usually take the train from Acton, and then the subway to Fenway Park. Unfortunately, late, on the way home, they ran into this large, maybe 350 pound bully. He accused the kids of laughing at him, and making fun of him. The parents of one of the kids just happened to be there, but they were too far away to see what was happening.

When the kids got off at their stop, the bully got off, too. When he was on the train, he said that he would "kick butt" when the kids got off. When they all got off, he kept stepping in front of the kids, blocking them, and pushing them around a bit. (Not David.) Some lady intervened, and told him to "back off." The bully and the woman started yelling at each other. This was enough of a distraction for the kids to slip away. Whew!

Friday, July 7

I'm sort of getting Peter ready for college. And I say, sort of, because he is such a procrastinator for things like that. He thinks, "Just throw a few things together a couple days before, and how hard can that be?" He reminds me of my brother, Jim, in so many ways. Peter leaves for Bucknell August 23. Kids take a lot more things these days than when I went to school.

Peter is still working 8-12 hours a day for a moving company, and besides, has his lawn business. Getting ready for school, being with friends, and just recently a girlfriend named Becky, all add up. I can see a clinging on to friends, as they all move toward that point of separation. It certainly leaves very little time for family life. Let's be honest—for me!!

David is busy growing up, up, up. In his spare time he works eight hours a day as a janitor's assistant at the high school, scraping gum off the bottom of desks, and other fun things. He also has a small lawn business, called Lawns for Less with his friend, Ron. (Not long after that, he expanded his lawn business with a partner, Eric. It was appropriately called The Lawn Crew, as they had several other kids working for them, their classmates. At the end of the year, David made a lobster dinner at the house, and also gave his workers bonuses. How keen is that!)

David and his friends went again last night to a Red Sox game. We, the parents, thought it best for the kids to take the subway again as soon as possible, even though David thought the bully would be waiting for them. I told David the odds were he would never be on the same car and at the same time ever again. The first time, the kids wreaked of suburbia with their Acton-Boxborough garb, so last night they dressed differently. The adults told them that they had to be "street smart," not joke around and laugh, and definitely, not stare at anyone. Basically, keep your eyes down. Everything turned out OK, and the Red Sox won 5-4.

I've been driving myself all around, and feeling comfortable, and also feeling I am quite good. I feel like a little girl who is getting away with something, or harboring some deep secret! It's great to have that independence, and not have to feel that I am imposing, or keeping someone waiting.

Some requests for résumés are drifting in. When my business cards are available, various shops will have them for distribution to the public. Employment agencies, colleges. The list is endless.

Tuesday, July 25

Today I saw Dr. Moore. I like seeing Dr. Moore, maybe because every time I go in there it is always "show and tell" time for me. He also does some basic neurological tests, and tells me how well I am doing. Following a little light with my eyes—do I see one or two? Then, a red light. Tapping my feet one at a time. Touching forefinger to thumb, both sides. I hate it when I have to do my right side, because my right is always slower, and this is a reminder to me (this test, this performance) I have a long way to go. I always say I am battling this and old age at the same time.

Next, test reflexes. Scratch the bottom of each foot with an instrument. (I could never understand when I was wearing nylon stockings, why they never ripped!) Walk tandem (placing one foot in front of the other heel to toe). I couldn't even do this, even before I got sick! Dr.Moore said I was walking much better. Most of the time, I know what the doctors are going to tell me, because I am very sensitive to my body, and how it is working. It is good to hear it from them, too, I must say.

Thursday, July 27

Drove to Burlington Mall today. Took David and his friend. Took the back roads, not the highway. Not confident going at a high rate of speed yet. I was really proud of myself. A 30-minute drive back in the dark, no less. I felt comfortable driving, and also comfortable walking in the mall. Not perfect, by a long shot, but I walked without the effort it took months ago. I feel my right leg lightening up, and my right side becoming more coordinated. It's been almost two years since my surgery, and I have "miles to go before I sleep."

Friday, July 28

I am pretty sensitive and aware of how I feel and why. Since I have been "sick," I have not had the least bit interest in men, that is, forming intimate relationships. Dr. V. said, "You're not weird. You are just handling a lot right now." But, I wonder. Perhaps, it is because of the "C" word. Perhaps to protect myself, I need to feel that way. Maybe, in the back of my mind, I am wondering no matter how great and strong I look, no matter what I say, no matter what great things I accomplish, no one may ever want to be with me. It may be too much of a risk for the other person. Then, again, everyone's life hangs on a thread. But, it just seems to me, that somehow it is different for people who have had a brush with death, or a struggle for life.

And, on another level, if a person were not interested simply because of my battle with cancer, I would seriously question that person's character and values, and then thank my lucky stars! If, on the other hand, another were truly interested, you might question that person's motive. It's all too complicated for me!

Sunday, August 13

David and I went out for some Chinese food. His fortune cookie read, "Someone will light up your life." Mine read, "Your weakness could be your strength." Hm-m-m-mm—Interesting!

This weekend Peter went to Martha's Vineyard with seven of his friends, including his girlfriend, Becky. Unfortunately, of all the weekends in the year, it rained Friday, Saturday, and today it is raining. I'm sure, even though a lot of their activities were curtailed, they had fun anyway.

Parents Weekend at Bucknell, Pennsylvania, is September 22, 23, 24. I already have plane reservations, and will be staying in a private home less than a mile from the campus. The owner of the house has offered to pick me up at the airport, and also give me rides back and forth to campus whenever I needed. I already reserved my same room for Spring Weekend in April. And even as ridiculous as it sounds, Bucknell strongly suggests parents make hotel reservations NOW for Commencement 1993.

Friday, August 18

I walked 5 miles. It was a nice coolish day, so I decided to take a short walk. But, I just kept walking and walking, and I said, "If I go around this way, that will make 4.3 miles, and if I go around once more that will make 5 miles." It's a record! Before this, it was 3.6 miles in sunny California, Christmas '88.

Saturday, August 19

Today the A-B Basketball Boosters had a bottle and can drive. First, David, his friend and I drove down our assigned streets to pick up any bags of bottles and cans which were placed at the end of driveways. Then to the junior high tennis courts to sort for seven hours. So many truckloads of bags back and forth to the store for refunds. The boosters made approximately $2,500; they were originally hoping to hit $1000. I was so happy I was able to be there. People asked me, "Aren't you tired?" I said, "No, it just bothers me if I have to move up and down a lot, because I get a little dizzy." It was a long time. I felt good that I was able to maneuver around the bags and hundreds of bottles stacked on the ground.

After that, a barbecue to celebrate. And after that, I went directly to a movie, "When Harry Met Sally," a story asking the question, "Can a man and a woman be just friends?" It was a last minute idea, and none of my friends were at home, so I went by myself. I enjoyed taking myself somewhere at night alone. Coming out of the movie, I was wondering if I would remember where I parked my car, or even if I could find it in the dark. No problem.

What a full day! I have so much energy that people are amazed. I guess I'm pretty amazed myself!

26.

THE EMPTYING OF THE NEST

Sunday, August 20

I wrote this letter to Peter today so he would receive it in his mailbox, upon his arrival to Bucknell University on the 23rd:

Dear Peter,

As you go off to school, I want to tell you that I am so happy and proud to have you as my son. You are strong and intelligent and kind, and a real pleasure, more than any mother could order, if she had her choice. I will miss your constant sense of humor, your integrity and stimulation. All of this will go with you to Bucknell, and many in your life will be enriched by these special qualities. I just have a few points I want to say. (OK, I'm getting the last word in!)

    1. Remember this in everything you do:

        God grant me the Serenity

        To Accept the things I cannot change;

The Courage to change the things I can,
And the Wisdom to know the difference.

2. Procrastination is deadly. More energy is consumed in procrastinating than in "getting it done". So, just do it!
3. Be true to yourself. If it feels right, it probably is.
4. "Take your time; don't move too fast; Troubles will come and they will pass." (Peter chose this quote for his senior photo in the yearbook)
5. Lestoil cleans almost anything.
6. I love you very much

Love,
Mom

Tuesday, August 22

The day before Peter leaves for school. Time for Peter to tie up some loose ends, go to the bank, etc. Oh yeah, maybe start packing! I have been piling things up in a corner of the dining room for some time now, and yesterday I committed the worst sin by going into Peter's room. I boxed up many years of Sports Illustrated magazines, organized his closet, and generally made a first attempt to break up dust particles and other matter.

Becky, his friend, took a half day off from work to help get on his case to pack. So, now it is 8:45 p.m. Peter was just beginning to pack the car, as his first bunch of friends stopped by. In came 20-25 friends to say goodbye. They sort of came in droves. They talked and laughed, exchanged college addresses, and watched TV. Amidst symbolic handshakes and farewell hugs, I saw a super connection, a camaraderie that is rare. There was happiness in their being together, but there was also sadness in their approaching separation. "When do you leave for school?" "I'm not a good letter writer." No matter. All summer long, it was "What are we doing tonight?" The process of separation started many months ago. There was a "clinging" and attempt to know friends even more, as each day passed.

I took a lot of pictures. By 10:45 p.m., they had all gone, and finally now, it was time for some serious packing. I lay on the couch, reading a book, feeling I had done all that I could at this point. I then fell asleep, and left the rest to Peter and Becky. At 12:45 a.m. I heard a voice say, "Ready for inspection,

Mom." And that is what I did. His small '76 BMW was packed like a can of sardines. I couldn't believe he got everything in, even though earlier he reassured me that he was a mover (his summer job) and that he could pack anything.

After that, morning came fast. It was time to go. The goodbye hug got to me, and I started crying. Peter said, "You don't have to cry just because you have to take over my dishes night!" The real heartbreaker was, when he was pulling out of the garage, he waved, and said, "I'll miss you." During the day, each time I told my friends about this, I would cry all over again!

An hour later, a friend asked me to go to the mall. I said, "This house is a mess, and I'm not finished crying, but I think I could probably pull myself together." After that, more errands, and then grocery shopping. I was exhausted and strained, but somehow today, I just had to keep moving.

Friday, September 1

I write Peter about every other day (I saved the letters and created a spiral–bound book out of them for a keepsake.), because I have so many details to tell him about, and local articles to send. When I talked to him on the phone, he said, "Mom, are you going to do this for four years?" I think he really likes getting the mail, and I'm sure I will taper off. But, it seems like I always have something to say or something to send. When I called last night, his roommate, Kirk, answered. All the guys in the hall had ordered out for pizza. He said, "Hey, everyone! Say hello to Pete's Mom", at which everyone chorused, "Hi Pete's Mom!" Today was the first day of classes at Bucknell, but Peter doesn't have any classes until Tuesday.

David didn't waste time moving his stereo, his clothes, and his body into Peter's room. He is enjoying the extra space, and it didn't take him long to take over Peter's portable phone. David had become Dave lately, and Peter became Pete a long time ago. Nobody calls them by their given names. (That's what you said would happen, Mom!) It's Bos, not Boswell (He has to go along with the kids.)

Saturday, September 2

I'm a little frustrated because I am right on the edge of getting "social" again, but I don't feel confident. Also, who wants to be with someone who has had cancer? That "C" word is scary, because the person might get it again. If a person has conquered cancer, that's great, but it is something one admires from a distance. To get close may be risky. It seems that the more I improve, the more I think about these kinds of things. For example, I'd love to go out dancing as I did before, but with someone who understands my situation. So, what is one to do?

27.

IN HIS EYES, FROM HIS HEART

Following is a paper David wrote for his English class assignment on November 20, 1988. The assignment was specifically to write about someone you admire. He decided to write about me, and he titled it "The Survivor." What a tribute from my son!

"After being through this brain cancer, I realize what it is like to be a baby, and also an elderly person", said my mom, a woman who has been through the ups and downs of life, as if she were a water skier. "Sometimes I feel like a baby because I am too uncoordinated to do some simple everyday things. Or, I feel like the elderly person, who is too old to move their bodies around, to do what normal people take for granted."

My mom is usually home day in and day out, after getting laid off from her job two years ago, and having been sick the past year and a half. Right now, with all of the leaves falling, she is usually outside raking, like there is no tomorrow. She straps on her work boots, and just rakes and rakes. "I like raking, because I know it is something that I can do." The neighbors see her out there raking every day, and they are just amazed! Their mouths are always wide open, when they see the day-to-day progress she is making.

"What do you guys want for dinner tonight?" is a question we hear almost every night. And, after dinner, we hear, "David, do you need help with the dishes?", when the kitchen looks like it has just been hit by a bomb. There are crumbled up napkins on the table, milk spilled on the table from my clumsy brother, plates filled with the remains of hamburgers and French fries; plus the dreadful cooking pan covered with grease and the bottoms of sticky hamburgers.

Whenever I come home from school or any extracurricular activity, you always hear, "How was school today? "How did you do on that English test?" or one of my soccer or basketball games, far more than any other parent. I remember during a basketball tournament, last winter, she went all the way to Bedford for every game, even when she could barely walk. She was at the game, slamming her cane down on the bleachers, as if she were some kind of barbarian, cheering as loud as her lungs would let her! It was almost as if she were in the game.

Even if she weren't at an event, my heart felt like she was there. The discipline that she instilled in me had stayed in my heart, and it always seems as though she is there, even when she isn't. All of those times that I heard "Clean your room, and make your bed," had paid off. At the time these commands did not seem fair, but I guess when you get older, you notice that the mother is always right. My mom has been through a lot of ups and downs in the past two years, but she has surpassed every one of them with flying colors.

28.

REFRIGERATOR POETRY

There are two pieces of poetry on my refrigerator that I would like to share. The papers are aged and brown. The first one was written January 23, 1978 by a young man, with whom I played in the theater. This is what he wrote and shared with the cast before he died of cancer.

THE GOOD SHIP LIVING

The good ship Living is for all to sail,
But, only a few do ever avail;
Energy and desire combine for the frame;
The sails are unique, never the same.

There are those who are the quest;
The voyage is Being; there is no rest;
Others are fearful, and remain at the gate;
The ship is before them, but they hesitate.

The ground is safe, and demands no change;
Sameness is everywhere, always within in range;
A choice exists for each, you see;
Sail the ship or endless security.

150

The voyage is not for a single mind,
Seek another who thinks in kind;
Set your sails quick, the wind blows to sea;
Time is short, the good ship is Destiny.

RISKS

"To laugh is to risk appearing the fool,
To weep is to risk appearing sentimental,
To reach out for another is to risk involvement,
To expose our feelings is to risk exposing our true self,
To place your ideas and dreams before a crowd is to risk loss,
To love is to risk not being loved in return,
To live is to risk dying,
To hope is to risk despair,
To try at all is to risk failure,
But, risk, we must, because the greatest hazard in life is to risk nothing.
The man, the woman, who risks nothing, does nothing, has nothing, is nothing."

29.

PERCEPTIONS—A CHANGE

Perceptions of certain words change, because I have changed. Words take on totally different meanings now. I will now describe the "**before**," the way I used to look at things, and the "**after**," the way I see things now.

PATIENCE

> **before:** Holding your temper; being tolerant of lines in the supermarket and other places.
> **after:** Being patient with the slowness of recovery of my neurological system; being tolerant of myself in holding lines up in the supermarket and other places.

COORDINATION

> **before:** Coordination, as in sports (i.e., Isn't that kid coordinated?)
> **after:** The loss of coordination, because of damage to the nervous system affecting writing (keep shoulder loose; don't hold the pen too tightly), personal grooming, dancing, driving, eating, walking, skipping, household chores, almost anything. Can't participate in sports. Catching a ball like a five year old, sort of flailing with the arms toward the chest, and closing the eyes. Viewing sports and dance and all activities involving coordination with more appreciation.

BALANCE

before: Balance beam in gymnastics, ballet, tightrope walker.

after: Not being able to walk or turn around smoothly. Can't wear high heel shoes or ride a bike. Impossible to try on clothes in a dressing room that does not have a stool.

WALK

before: Go for a walk through the woods; something pleasant to do.

after: A real privilege, a miracle that we take for granted. A workout; concentration. What's causing my staggering? Do I need to take longer strides? Am I thrusting my hip forward enough? Arms swinging. Torso loose. Walk in the center of the foot; don't slap it down. Hard work. When walking, stop before looking to either side, or you will stagger. Keep working at walking, until it becomes fun. I realize how much the condition of my eyes affects my walking.

FUN

before: Seeing friends, dancing, dinner, movie, theater (as a performer and a spectator). Beach. Club Med vacations. Going to my kids' activities.

after: Seeing friends, dancing (I'm getting there!). Going to my kids' activities, accomplishing new things every day, feeling more independent, managing the street curbs all by myself.

HANDICAPPED

before: Someone in a wheelchair, or with a disease; physically or mentally impaired; handicapped parking spaces. Dependent. Unfortunate. Not me.

after: Me. Dependent. Shower bar and shower chair. Wheelchair and walker and cane. Hand railings. People to do all my shopping and cleaning, and take care of me. Drivers to take me to do my errands, when I was able to go along. Always feeling like I am being hauled around, even though my friends are very kind and helpful.

HURRY

before: Rushing to get a job done at work or at home, rushing to get to work or an appointment, or pick up the kids. Rushing to get groceries, rushing to have fun. In Arabic, it sounds like "yell-ah".

after: What, me worry? What, me hurry? Can't.

FRIEND

before: Someone who shares your joys and sorrows. Someone you trust.

after: Someone who sticks with you through "thick and thin." Someone who is patient with your changes.

PROBLEM

before: Not getting enough done in a day, crossing off "to do" list items. Disagreeing with a supervisor, whom I felt was unfair or less intelligent than I, but finding myself in the less powerful position.

after: Not doing things fast enough. Dropping things more. Not able to do things with ease, such as climbing steps, turning hamburgers, sewing, walking, stepping in and out of the shower, getting up in the morning, knowing I have to continue to struggle to get better, all day long, with everything.

PRAYER

before: The telephone line, the communication line, between people and God. An act of faith. For most people, mostly done at church, and off and on at other places. More during times of trouble. The Lord's Prayer. Praying for others.

after: If prayer were telephone calls, my bill would be astronomical! People praying for me all over Massachusetts, all over the world. The words "I'll pray for you" take on a deeper meaning. You realize you are a human being, and prayer is it.

NOISE

before: At a competitive sports game. Loud music. Loud talking in a small room. Dog barking.

after: *All* sounds became more pronounced and very bothersome. In the beginning, a utensil dropping on the floor. The closing of a door, a dripping faucet. I have some friends who don't have the softest of voices, but I wanted to be with them. And sometimes they would have to drive me places. So, I had to ignore my extreme sensitivity to their voices be with them.

STRESS

before: Working well and hard at my job, but not being appreciated or compensated. Rushing to get home from work to pick up someone, somewhere, on time. Trying to get everything done on the weekend, that I couldn't get done during the week. Trying to take a little time for myself by being in the theater and doing yoga. Finding out, that even though this was good for me, I was still stressed out trying to balance everything.

after: Having brain cancer. O-o-oh, those dirty words! Bad enough having cancer, but brain cancer! Double O-o-oh. More like, uh–oh! Chemotherapy. Radiation. All the times in-between. Having so many people depend on you to get better. The daily grind. The daily discipline. Dealing with my own high expectations of myself and my limitations. It is hard being me. Trying to be the best single mother I can possibly be.

SEX/ATTRACTION

before: Interested. Having those unbelievable thrilling feelings. Passion.

after: Not interested. More a passion for walking, for life, becoming more independent. Not going outside of myself to attain a certain feeling or happiness. Not depending on that.

TIME

before: Never having enough time to do what I have to do.

after: Time is valuable. Life is short. People spend too much time bickering about unimportant things, and dwelling on small differences that should be put way down on the priorities list. Tolerance for each other's idiosyncrasies. Continually understanding and adjusting to one another.

LOVE

before: That deep trust in someone, who understands your changes, and allows you to be yourself. Husband, wife, lover, child, parent, friend, even dog.

after: Same feeling, except more, and deeper.

WHAT'S HAPPENIN'?

before: What's going on? New dress? Where did you get it? What movie? Was it good? Where did you go? What are you doing?

after: How are your eyes? Doctors' appointments. Therapy sessions. Walking so many miles with my cane, without my cane. Progress reports.

MIRACLE

before: Stories you read in the Bible about healing, or see on TV, especially the true stories of people who have beat the odds.

after: I am told, it is I.

FAMILY

before: Institution. Nuclear family (mother, father, and children, or in my case, just mother and children) and my extended family in California. All close, loving.

after: The strength of a family, as a unit, being tested. None as tough or as loving as mine. Nor as kind and caring, and I have to add to this—smart!

CONFIDENCE

before: Finally gaining confidence as a mother, in my career, on the stage.

after: Confidence is shot. Dependence does that. When a person is stripped of her identity, or what she knew herself to be, confusion results. The person can't depend on herself, because when she gets sick, or has something taken away, then that person has to get to know herself all over again. This takes time, as confidence builds on little successes. And confidence builds on confidence.

X-RAY

before: Check for broken bones. Dental X-rays. Chest X-ray.

after: CAT Scan every three months. MRI. Why didn't the tumor show up in the beginning? Why do some women discover they have breast cancer after their mammograms showed negative?

SELF-ESTEEM

before: How a person feels about herself. Intelligent. Professional. Good mother. Attractive 40's. Passionate. Good dancer.

after: Fat, bald, and ugly. Slow. Body not able to keep up with mind. Clumsy. Forgetful. Not a good feeling.

PRIORITIES

before: Kids and friends and family. Job. Cleaning. Laundry.

after: Me first, or else I can't do anything, or help anyone. Just as the airlines instruct their passengers—the oxygen mask goes first on the adult, and then on the child. I am not much use to anyone, unless I take care of myself, and get better. It I can learn something along the way, this would be an extra benefit.

HELPLESS

before: A baby who needs to be fed, changed. Dependent on adults, especially the first year of life.

after: Like a baby. Dependent on others. No matter how much you want to do something, no matter how much your mind says, "Do it," if your body is not in sync with your mind, it won't happen. For, example, you feel helpless if you want to get up, but can't.

FRUSTRATION

before: Not being able to get enough things done in a day. As in my college psychology course, a book titled, "Frustration Leads to Aggression."

after: Caused by helplessness; no control.

SUBMISSION

before: Opposite of powerful. Cowering. An employee toward an employer. A submissive wife. A dependent role.

after: Do what you want with me. Take a blood sample. Get me the bedpan. Wheel me around. Take out my brain. I don't care because I'm too sick, weak and dependent.

DOCTOR'S APPOINTMENT

before: Check up; pap smear.

after: Follow-up on tumor. Neurological exam. Walk around the table. What's new since the last time? The list of good things or accomplishments; the list of bad things or frustrations. See you in three months.

VICTORY

before: A win in sports.

after: "You're our little victory. You're our inspiration." Being successful with yourself. Being true to yourself. Reaching for your potential. One reason I feel that I have to keep getting well is because others believe in me. Many people have supported me with their prayers and in many other ways, and I don't want to let them down. I also feel that I will be victorious in this battle. As I said to Dr. Tripp, my children's pediatrician, in intensive care, "I have a lot more living to do; I have a lot more to give." I remember that.

30.

AUBREY

Aubrey. It is hard to describe Aubrey. Harder than the Mona Lisa. My mother said, "Where did this man come from?" A gift from God. Our children were best friends in school, so he wanted to be my friend. After a couple of times together, I got sick. And, after I was diagnosed with Multiple Sclerosis, I told him he'd better run, that "this was not the flu." He never left. He spent many hours at the hospital, and many hours driving me and my mother to hospitals and doctors. Much later on, shopping or out to lunch, or any place I needed to go. Also, he gave rides to my kids when needed, and bought groceries and did laundry. He also bought me an answering machine, so I wouldn't miss any important calls.

He came every night to make sure I had juices and a banana or other food next to the couch or bed. He made sure my walker was within my reach, as it had to be exact to prevent me from falling. He let the dog in, and made sure all appropriate lights were on or off before he went home. When I finally was able to move upstairs to my bedroom, he followed me up with my goodies, and tucked me in.

He always made sure I had fresh flowers.

He creamed my legs in the hospital, and also shaved my legs when I got home. (He knew how much I hated hairy legs!) I was unable to groom myself. One time he shaved my legs with the cover still on the razor. We thought this was pretty funny!

He walked the streets of Boston with my mom, to try to find a pharmacy that would take my insurance card. Otherwise, we would have had to pay $400 for nine doses! (Note: Presently, 2001, those same pills are $72 each!)

Aubrey was always there for me anytime, anywhere. Pretty soon, it became a big joke, "Did he ever go to work?"

Sometimes he was too protective, and didn't realize that I had done something by myself that day. So, occasionally, I had to let him know.

When I was "fat, ugly, and bald", he didn't see what I saw. He knew how much I hated how I looked. He always gave me encouragement, and told me I was pretty, even when I knew I wasn't. Sometimes he called me "Pretty."

Here is a man who carried me down the steps in my nightgown. He walked me to the hospital bathroom, when I was clad only in a "johnny." He shaved my legs, and watched me brush my teeth. Even though there was no "intimacy," as most people know it, we had more. Our friendship has such depth and character, which words defy to describe. Like a seed that grows. Or a building with a strong foundation. With the ease of a flowing river, or the opening of a rose petal. This is how I feel it to be.

As I improved, adjustments had to be made. As I gained more independence, I needed more privacy. So, not only did I have to adjust to my own progress, and increased confidence, but I had to be aware of everyone else having to adjust, too. Friends and neighbors who were used to doing everything for me, had to adjust to not being needed as much. Ironically, at times I had to help wean them from tending to me, so I would ask them for a favor. On the other hand, I'm sure there were others who had better things to do.

I felt I had a meter inside of me that sort of gauged my progress. And I had to continuously do a reading, and let everyone know where I stood. Since Aubrey was my main support, there had to be a lot of consistent communication. I am sure this understanding and sensitivity on both parts, is what has made us such special friends.

No doubt about it. Aubrey is a loving, caring, and very special man, and I am a lucky, lucky lady.

✳ ✳

At the time I am writing this addition (January 1990), our relationship has changed. I have improved considerably, and naturally I have become less dependent on others. Although this independence has lead to a feeling of freedom for me, it has resulted in one of abandonment for Aubrey. It seems that when I was depending on him, he was also depending on me, as obviously, he was playing a major role in someone else's life.

31.

DON'T ASK "WHY ME?"

I never asked why. I never asked, "Why me?" because there is no answer. We never know the reason why certain bad things happen. Or why does that happen? Why does this person have to suffer or die? When one survives, people say, "God was with you," but, if you die,.......? I believe we have no control over when we die—only God does. But, we *do* have control in how we *handle* a situation or crisis, whether it be in the process of living or dying. I believe that things sometimes happen for reasons beyond our control. Perhaps we are put in certain situations, and lead down different paths, because we are meant to touch certain lives or they, ours. The enrichment of lives may not be revealed for years, and may also last for generations. It is not for the mortal being to know or ask why.

"Fadel tough" That's what we call it. My mother always said, "When you get knocked down, get up, dust yourself off, and try again. You have to roll with the punches." Everyone gets punched. Different ways. Different places. Different times. But, we all get it.

Some professional people told me, "You'll never be the same again." They're right about that one. I'm a much better person. Needless to say, I have a new perspective on life. I'm more understanding, patient, tolerant of people—old people, handicapped people, children (and how they grow and develop), and others who have to deal with life's daily stresses and obstacles.

I have been forced to slow down, and become more organized, so that I can accomplish everything. I had to deal with the frustration of my mind racing ahead of my body. I know how the elderly must feel who have to deal with this phenomenon.

Someone asked me, "Did the tumor affect your memory?" I said, "Yeah, it made it better!" For example, I found that since my coordination was affected, that it was much easier for me to remember things, than to reach for a pen and write them down.

A neighbor's young son very insightfully said to me, "Mrs. Jepsen, I'll bet you learned a lot, and that you have a different perspective on life." I said, "Yes, you're right, Ron John, but I wouldn't want to do it again!" And I ask myself, "Would you trade places with anyone else?" The answer is "No." Of course, I want to walk more normally, and run, and drive and work, and do so many things. But, I wouldn't want to have someone else's life. I am so blessed with two great sons, the most beautiful mother in the world, two special sisters and a brother, and friends who are true blue—other people would die for. Add my dog, Boswell, who only digs trenches on his side of the yard. What more can a person ask for than all of this? I guess I am just plain lucky! We all have to play with the cards that are dealt to us. These words taken from the song, "The Gambler" says it all:

"Every gambler knows
That the secret to survivin'
Is knowin' what to throw away,
And knowin' what to keep...

Every hand's a winner,
And every hand's a loser...
You gotta know when to hold 'em,
Know when to fold 'em.
Know when to walk away,
Know when to run;

You never count your money
While you're sittin' at the table;
There'll be time enough to count,
When the dealin's done."

32.

MY WORST FEAR—
THE UNEXPECTED

On March 4, 1997, I moved from Massachusetts to sunny California, away from my doctors, including Dr. Hochberg at Mass General Hospital in Boston, my health insurance, and my best friends. The diagnosis of my first cancer was August 26, 1987, so I am now cancer-free for nine and a half years. What do people say, "After passing the critical five-year-period, that's it. You made it. You're cured." Hold your horses, partner, not so fast!

It felt as if one moment I was doing fine, and soon I was not. I realized something was not quite right, how I started losing a thought in mid-sentence and how my walking became visibly unstable. Twelve years ago when I was diagnosed with Cerebellum Lymphoma, my mother asked Dr. Amy Pruitt how we would know if my cancer might be returning. She said I would be the first to know from my walking and other signs.

You might think that I had a clue when my cancer was returning when my walking became more unstable with time. I just denied it, I guess. Though neighbors pulled aside in their cars to ask me why I was limping, I simply said, "This is the way I walk." One day a security officer in my village named Clyde, stopped and got out of his car. He said, "Are you all right?" I said, "Yes, why?" He said, "Because you are staggering." I replied, "I always stagger!"

After numerous visits to doctors in California for neurological and eye problems, with the only result being confused and frustrated doctors, I decided to go back to Massachusetts to see Dr. Fred Hochberg, a world-renown neuro-oncologist. He was key in saving my life when he diagnosed me with Cerebellum Lymphoma, 12 years ago.

At that time, there was the option of two treatments. If I (my Mom) would have chosen the "regular treatment", the doctor said I would live one year. With the experimental treatment of Methotrexate chemotherapy and high doses of radiation, he did not know how much longer I would live. And so the latter was chosen for me by my Mom. Twelve years later, the same Methotrexate chemotherapy was given to me, but in triple doses.

My health insurance in California would pay for my medical expenses in Massachusetts through a "guesting" policy provided by my health insurance, requiring I stay at least three months. I really did not know if I would be able to stay for three months, because three months away from home is a long time. Turns out, I had no choice. Instead, I stayed over five months with a few days back to California in-between.

This is my story.

Monday, August 16, 1999

I flew to Massachusetts where I stayed with my son, David, and his girlfriend, Gina, and a Golden Retriever, Gretsky. I stayed there for a couple days, and then went to my friend, Fran's house, where I stayed about three weeks.

One night (about 9:15 p.m.), when I was in my bedroom on the second floor and Fran was in the basement watching TV, I discovered I could not speak. I tried saying "David," to myself, but the word would not come out. I tried saying my name, but the best thing that came out was gibberish sounds. I then tried to write a list for the next day, but that was a problem, and I could not do that either. All I could manage were little scratches, no letters. I was puzzled and scared, but I was surprised how calm I was, and how I took mental account of what was happening and what time it was.

About 9:30 p.m., I went downstairs crying (I didn't have a problem doing that!). Somehow I encouraged Fran to talk to me and ask me questions that I might be able to answer. At first, she asked me a question, but I could not speak. As I motioned for her to continue, I could see in her face an anxious beckoning for me to try to speak. Finally, I did, and I was afraid to stop, for fear I would not talk again. Fran then offered to take me to the ER at Emerson

Hospital, in Concord. I probably should have gone, but I told Fran I was too tired, so I went the next morning to see my neurologist, Dr. Michael Moore in the John Cuming Building connected to the hospital. He admitted me from his office.

Wednesday, September 1

First office visit with my CIGNA primary care doctor, Dr. Gregory Martin, Concord Hillside Medical Center in Concord, whom I had never met before.

Tuesday, September 7

Office visit with neurologist, Dr. Michael Moore.

Wednesday, September 8

Moved from Fran's house to the Melia family's house.

Wednesday, September 15

EMG (tube down throat to heart) at Emerson Hospital to determine if there was a problem with my heart, or a possible TIA (transient-ischemic attack or mini-stroke). This test was given to possibly find out why I had lost my speaking and writing abilities. Dr. Boffetti, cardiologist, diagnosed that a piece of plaque got loose from the artery and went to the brain. He put me on Cumadin (blood thinner), which I took until a week before my eye biopsy (victrectomy) on November 12. I have not taken it since. Turned out later, this was all part of the unknown cancer of five tumors lurking in my brain!

Monday, September 20

Appointment with Dr. Moore, neurologist.

Wednesday, September 22

Appointment with Dr. Martin, primary care physician.

Friday, September 24

Office visit with ophthalmologist, Dr. Paul Vinger, to examine eyes for problem since January, 1997. Diagnosis: vitreous detachment (same diagnosis I have been getting all along, including uveitis). Prescribed new glasses.

Monday, September 27

CAT Scan. Picked up old MRI from Emerson Hospital in Concord for comparison at Massachusetts General Hospital in Boston.

Tuesday, September 28

Picked up new glasses from Gordon Optical in Concord.

Wednesday, September 29

First office visit with Dr. Fred Hochberg, neuro-oncologist in the Cox Building #315, Mass General Hospital. My son, David, was all set to take me, but he hurt his back, so his girlfriend, Gina, drove to Acton where I was staying with the Melia family and took me to see Dr. Hochberg.

As we sat in his office, he asked Gina if she knew me a long time, because he wanted to ask her questions about the possible changes in my speech. Of course, she said no. At the end of the appointment he recorded his report into a tape recorder. His first sentence was: "Dear Diane, When I saw you on the 29th of September, it was with the knowledge that you are probably the longest survivor of brain lymphoma in the United States." Gina and I just looked at each other shocked in amazement!

Gina also had an appointment with her doctor at the hospital for a lump under her arm, but it turned out to be an ingrown hair ("whew!"). We walked back to her and David's apartment on Beacon Hill. I just held on to her arm or purse strap to steady myself. She wanted to check on David and see if he needed anything. We walked, as their apartment was close to the hospital, and parking was scarce around their apartment.

I immediately loved this young woman for her love, her strength, her compassion, her ways of thinking, and her dedication to my son. She didn't stop here with her support. What else could I ask for in a woman who was soon to be engaged to my son?

Friday, October 1

Called for referral for Digitrace (48 hour computerized monitor) to determine if there were any serious neurological problems.

Thursday, October 14

My friend, Valerie, took me to this crazy appointment. About 18 electrodes were glued to my head. Gauze was then wrapped around my head and under my chin. I looked as if I had a head injury from a car accident or something. I had Valerie take pictures of the whole process, because when would this ever happen again??!!!

The wires on the electrodes were attached to a fanny-pack type computer, with a button that I would push if I felt the least abnormal neurological feelings. This was connected to the main computer that sat on the floor, and was plugged into the wall. (Get the picture?) If I had to go to the bathroom or whatever, I would pull the plug from the wall, and the computer on my waist would take over. However, most of the time I had to be plugged into the wall; I only was permitted to push the button so many times when I was unplugged.

Valerie took me back to the Melia's house where I was residing in an apartment on the second floor. To be close to the phone, I decided to sleep on the couch.

The saga continues!

Disaster of all disasters. One night at 2 a.m., my whole entire gauze "hat" fell off my head, with the wires dangling. I didn't want to bother Ann, especially at this hour, so I called the 24 hour Digitrace number. However, they had to call me back, and so therefore, woke up Ann and her husband. Thinking something might be wrong, he suggested his wife go upstairs to check on me. After examining the situation, she got her son's wool cap, gathered all my electrode wires, and stuffed them into the cap. I could not resist having a picture of this, too!

The Melia family is one of the finest, loving, caring families on God's earth. Not only did they take care of me, and give me rides to my many appointments, but invited me for dinner every night. Ann consistently cooked a variety of nutritious meals. It was exciting to sit around the table with the family as they talked about their sons' sports and activities at their individual schools, and also professional teams. In addition, there was talk about their two daughters who were making their way in the world. I can't say enough about Ann—about the rare kind of mother, wife and friend she is, and how she was sensitive to my every need.

Tuesday, October 19

First office visit with ophthalmologist/specialist Dr. Delia Sang (pronounced "song"), Beacon Street, Brookline, who is the "Dr. Hochberg of ophthalmology". She was very knowledgeable, thorough, energetic, and very quickly suspected lymphoma in my eyes. She liked wearing red and she was very cute with her small black fanny pack she always wore. It was a trademark. What did she carry in it? Probably keys and tissue like everyone else! Scheduled an eye biopsy (vitrectomy) for November 12.

Thursday, October 21

Dr. Henry Vaillant, my former primary care physician for over 20 years, a co-worker at Acton Medical Center, and a friend, asked me out to lunch. However, I did not feel well enough, so I made him a grilled cheese sandwich. He said it was the best grilled cheese sandwich he had ever had in his life! He entered the apartment through a separate entrance on the side of the house. When he entered, he handed me a twig he got from a plant outside Acton Medical Center (where his office is), planted by doctors years ago. I forgot the name of the plant with the orange-type berries. As he went down the steps, I yelled to him, "What does this mean?" He turned his head upward and said, "It's a healing branch." I adore Dr. Vaillant! Everyone does.

Saturday, October 22

This was the night of Ann's birthday party at the Colonial Inn in Concord. Kevin, Ann's husband, invited me to go, but I declined, as I did not want to take the attention away from Ann on her special day.

About 2:30–3 p.m., I was running from my bed to catch the phone in the next room. I lost my balance, listing to the right, hit the angled wall, and propelled myself to the left, falling with excruciating pain. As I never got to the phone, the younger son answered the phone downstairs, and said it was for me. The message was that my friend, Mary, who was going to pick me up at 5 p.m. to go to her mother's house for dinner, was coming one hour earlier at 4 p.m. How lucky could I get? I yelled to the son for help. I told him I was OK, and to tell my friend I would return the call. He thought I was fine and never appeared again. This is a big house, and it is hard to be heard if you are in another room.

I crawled to the refrigerator, and lucky for me there was a cold pack in the freezer. I then crawled to the phone to make a call, but one of the daughters was on the line downstairs. I interrupted her call, and told her I needed help. She came upstairs right away. She sat next to me and asked me if I wanted her to take me to the emergency room. I declined because that would take hours, and I did not want her to miss her mother's party.

It soon became 4 p.m., and Mary appeared to take me to her mother's house—so she thought. Instead, I made some sort of a sling with my wool scarf. Then she gently and slowly helped me down the steps and into her car to go to the emergency room. I don't know how we did that! She stayed with me for hours. The X-ray showed a fractured left clavicle. This was all I needed, and this was all the Melia family needed!

I am here in Massachusetts for unsolved neurological problems, and now I have a broken bone! The hospital set me up with a sling that was pretty much useless, because it kept slipping off.

Shortly after this fiasco, my dear friend, Ann, realized that I was too sick and unstable to stay with her, as she could no longer meet my needs. She was direct, but said it in the kindest way possible. I then went to a rehabilitation nursing home near Emerson Hospital. I was there only one day, because I was so upset with my terrible treatment there.

I called my son, David, to pick me up, and Gina came with him. He thought maybe I should stay because it was a convenient place to be, until I told him what a nightmare it was for me. Didn't take me long to figure that out! I stayed with him and Gina in their apartment (very small) for two days. We then decided that maybe the best thing would be for me to return to California for treatment. David made special arrangements with the airlines, and then I was off.

Saturday, October 30

I flew back to California, hoping to be treated on my home turf, with direction from Dr. Hochberg to California doctors. In the meantime, Georgia, my sister, who lived in the San Francisco area, called Dr. Hochberg immediately. He told her my case was too complicated to be treated in California, and that I needed to return to Massachusetts as soon as possible.

I really had no choice. Because of the critical timing involved, the Massachusetts doctors told me that I would not have survived if I stayed in California, as I did not have my doctors and other medical personnel lined up.

Whereas, in Massachusetts, twelve years ago, the doctors knew my history with brain cancer, and were therefore ready for me. Georgia took hours and days to finally arrange through Mass General Hospital Social Services a place for us to stay. She met me at our mother's house. (I could not go to my house because I had rented it out for the few months that I was going to be in Massachusetts.)

Monday, November 8

Georgia and I flew back to Boston to a place for us at the YMCA Constitution Inn, sponsored by Mass General for patients and their families. It was a difficult journey because I was becoming increasingly unstable.

Tuesday, November 9

MRI (Magnetic Resonance Imaging) at Mass General Charlestown facility. Since the facility was walking distance from our inn, Georgia pushed me in a wheelchair to the appointment.

Wednesday, November 10

Office visit with Dr. Hochberg, mainly to hear the results of the MRI. Georgia and I took the shuttle to the hospital. He walked into the room looking not so happy. I picked up on this right away, and said to him, "I don't like how you look." He told Georgia and me the MRI showed I had five lesions in my brain. Georgia asked, "What is the difference between lesions and tumors?" He said, "They are the same."

He looked down and said, "I can't tell you how distressed I am!" He proceeded to give us some facts. "I am not sure what we will treat the tumors with because I can't use Methotrexate twice since you used it twelve years ago when you had Cerebellum Lymphoma. You will have to stay here at the minimum three months."

He looked at Georgia and asked, "Can you stay?" and Georgia responded, "I can't stay three months!" He said, "If not, Diane may as well fly home with you tomorrow!" He gave us until the next day to make a decision. He then got up, left the room, while our heads started buzzing with thoughts. He had a student there with him from Germany, Eva, who tried to comfort us, and help us figure out housing, etc.

As Dr. Hochberg was leaving the room, Georgia instinctively started to follow him to ask more questions, but he told her he couldn't talk right now, and left the building. Dr. Chioria came in and said Dr. Hochberg went home because he was sick. It didn't take more than a few minutes for Georgia and I to know we were both staying in Boston. Georgia did not want to take the shuttle back home to our place, so she called David at work. Then David called Gina, who was at the apartment. Before David arrived, Gina ran to the hospital lobby to meet us.

Keep your eyes focused on Georgia. Just call her Tiny, but Mighty!

Thursday, November 11

Office visit with Dr. Sang, day before biopsy. David and Gina picked Georgia and me up from the Constitution Inn. I was so weak they all had to help me into the car.

Friday, November 12

To Mass Eye and Ear for biopsy of right eye, which was a success, showing eye lymphoma. This was followed by many eye drops and ointment which had to be given at specific times, sometimes minutes apart. Dr. Sang did not want to schedule me for radiation for my eyes for six weeks after the biopsy.

Saturday, November 13

Saw Dr. Sang at Mass Eye and Ear. She was very pleased and said my eye looked "fabulous"! She liked using that word, and I liked hearing it! Off to the pharmacy to fill many prescriptions.

When Georgia and I returned to the Constitution Inn, my speech was even more slurred, and my balance was rapidly deteriorating. Since arriving on Monday, I had gone from bad to worse. In the beginning, Georgia set up chairs leading to the bathroom, so I would have something to hold on to. By Saturday, Georgia was taking me to the bathroom with barely enough strength to hold me up. Before bedtime, Georgia knew I needed to be in the hospital.

Sunday, November 14

Georgia then called Dr. Hochberg, but talked to the on-call neurologist, who said he and Dr. Hochberg would be in a meeting, and he would give him the message. When there was no response for an hour, Georgia called again and said, "If Dr. Hochberg does not call, I will admit my sister myself! I'm bringing her in right now!" Dr. Hochberg called back in five minutes.

Immediately, she heard he was confused. He was told the wrong name, Diane Jackson, instead of Diane Jepsen.

Georgia then called David to tell him I was weak, and she needed his help to take me to the hospital. David and Gina, both came immediately. David's sports car was too small, so we jumped (Jump? Not I!) into a taxi. I didn't understand why I had to go to the hospital, because I didn't think I was *that* sick.

That evening Dr. Chioria, a colleague of Dr. Hochberg, showed a copy of the MRI to Georgia, David and Gina. The doctor thought thatMethotrexate wouldn't work, because as Dr. Hochberg had mentioned, that was used on me twelve years ago, and it maybe would cause dementia. He said that the only other treatment left was Topotecan, a new chemotherapy that started at Mass General. So far, they had only used it on nine patients. Three had survived, and one was presently on this treatment. If it didn't work, I would have approximately two months to live. Georgia did not put a lot of weight on what he said, because it was not Dr. Hochberg speaking. She would wait to hear Dr. Hochberg's recommendations.

Monday, November 15

Dr. Hochberg came into my room and said to Georgia and me. "I've been thinking of this all night, and this is what I have decided: We will use Methotrexate in about triple the dose of what you had twelve years ago. Since you are the only survivor of this type of tumor, treatment has never been tried with a twelve-year break between treatments. As it was twelve years ago, this will be experimental. He also said "Diane, you are very sick and you could die," to which I responded heartily, "You could die, too!"

From then on, Georgia was with me at the hospital every day, from breakfast until after dinner, kind of running the whole show. In the beginning, she was there to feed me and brush my teeth. (Please see the two page article that appeared in the Massachusetts General Hospital's newsletter dated April 20, 2000 later in this manuscript.) By now, my sister is the main caretaker of me, my meds and my entire well-being. She soon got a reputation with the nurses and doctors alike. A favorite nurse, named Adelle, told me, "Georgia has given us strict orders about the frequency of the drops."

The head doctor in radiation at Mass General wanted to treat my eyes with radiation right away. However, Dr. Sang's orders were to wait at least six weeks after the biopsy. Georgia had a heated discussion with the doctor. She told Georgia that she knew more about radiation than Dr. Sang or Dr. Hochberg, and that I should be treated now. She told Georgia, "Do you want your sister to go blind?" Georgia responded, "You are not to touch my sister unless you ask me, and Dr. Sang and Dr. Hochberg say OK." Georgia immediately called Dr. Sang and let her know what the radiation doctor said. Dr. Sang, in turn, called Dr. Hochberg, who was out of town on a seminar. He returned home one day early because of the radiation situation. He called Georgia and apologized because the doctor was trying to intimidate her. Of course, the end result was, we waited to have the radiation treatment.

I soon was sent to the radiation department for preparation only. They took a wet piece of plastic-like grid material and molded it to my face. This was used during radiation, as they had to keep my head still by clamping down on the mask that was formed. (Presently, I have this mask hanging on my bedroom wall with a collection of other various masks.) Anyway, when I finally went for my treatment, I saw about 30 other masks lined up, which were labeled for other patients. That was quite a sight! What a photo that would have made!

Georgia left the room for a few minutes, and when she got back, I was not there. A nurse told her I went to radiation. Georgia said, "Somebody go get her right now, or I am going to get her myself! Nobody takes my sister without asking me first!" Noreen Leahy, Dr. Hochberg's nurse practitioner, checked and told Georgia, "She just went to radiation to get fitted for a mask."

Georgia knew Dr. Sang wanted to wait for about six weeks, and somebody in radiation had contested her on that, and she was afraid they sneaked me out of my room. Georgia told Dr. Sang that the person in radiology said she knew more than Dr. Sang. What do you think Dr. Sang said about that? Georgia was not going to let anybody do anything without Dr. Sang's orders. How would you like to have a sister as smart and strong as this one on your side?

Monday, November 16

Georgia moved to the Beacon House, also run by Mass General Hospital for patients and their families. Stayed there until November 29. She then moved to an apartment on Beacon Hill for $1900 a month. She wanted to have a place close to the hospital, and also a larger place ready for me, in case I had to have a caretaker stay with me full-time. That never happened, I needed no help when I moved in. (more later)

Tuesday, November 17

When a patient is having chemotherapy, a warning sign is put on the door, and the nurses wear thick blue gloves when they are handling the chemo and urine. The following description of the process may not be totally accurate.

The start of my first Methotrexate chemotherapy. Each treatment is a process which I will try to explain as accurately as I can:

- First, a 24-hour urine collection must be taken to test the alkaline/acid.
- Blood needs to be drawn at the lab.
- Biocarbonate pills (20) need to be taken throughout the day before chemo begins.
- Upon arrival to my room at the hospital the portacath in my chest needs to be accessed. When this is being done, sometimes I have to wear a mask as the nurse or turn my head away, so I don't breathe on the portacath. Sometimes, the nurses have a hard time accessing, so I am asked either to sit up or cough. Sometimes they have to try a longer needle.
- Pre-hydration by IV for six hours. When urine and blood levels are appropriate, the Methotrexate is started which takes approximately four hours. This can be started at any time, even in the wee hours of the morning, depending on the levels.
- For the rest of time while I am there (whole process takes over three days) urine is measured and tested almost every single time.
- Then I am hydrated for hours.
- Next, comes four cycles of IV Calcium Leukovorin (six hours apart with hydration in-between), which is an antidote to the Methotrexate. By some miracle to me, it takes the Methotrexate out of the good cells and leaves it to tackle bad cells. (or takes it out of the body and leaves it in the brain.)
- When I return home, I need to continue taking Calcium Leucovorin in pill form for nine doses every six hours, which means setting the alarm. If not done on time, the result could be fatal.

When my urine and blood levels are appropriate, I am ready to go home. The nurse de-accesses the needles from the portacath. *I am free!* The night before discharge, I have already started packing all my stuff! Clothes (I don't wear johnnies), books, important papers, blank paper, pens, telephone numbers, hormone therapy pills, etc., etc., even before I am de-accessed, because I am so excited. I so much look forward to going home to resume my normal activities and eating when and what I wish.

One of the toughest things about chemo treatments is being limited, as you are connected to an IV pole, which becomes part of you, even as you go to the bathroom or take a walk down the hall. You are totally dependent on your nurses, and if you are unable to go to the bathroom by yourself, this can be tough. Scenario: You ring the nurse button, but they are all busy, and might not get to you before you wet your bed. Since you have some kind of liquid going into you the entire time, you are constantly having that urge to go to the bathroom. Also, unfortunately for me, chemo brought on constipation and loss of appetite.

Two times I got sick the last fifteen minutes of the actual four-hour Methotrexate IV treatment. Gina is a nurse in the cardiac department at Mass General, and was working, when she saw a lot of chaos and commotion in my room through a window across the way. (She knew it was my room because I had a lot of flowers in my window) The nurses were scurrying around me, because I had just vomited all over the place. Gina had no idea what was happening, so she excused herself from her job to check on me.

Huge improvements in my speech were especially noticeable after my first chemo.

I did everything possible to become as independent as I possibly could. I had to convince the nurses that I was able to transfer myself to the commode next to the bed. How did I do this? I enlisted physical therapy to teach me.

Weeks later there was a "code blue" emergency announcement to Ellison 12 (Ellison Building, 12th floor). I was on this floor. Gina was one of the nurses who rushed to this floor. Once again, she was concerned the emergency might have been me, but it was the man next door. He died. (When someone dies, they close all the patients' doors.)

More than once when Gina had worked those thirteen hour shifts, she would come to see me before she went home. She was so tired, so I would invite her to lie on top of my bed with me. We would lie there and watch TV and eat chocolates. (Those truffles were yummy, right Gina?!)

I soon learned that the nurses checked your status every day: "Do you know what day it is? OK, right! There was a calendar on the wall!) "What is your name?" "Where are you?" "Who is the President of the United States?" Pretty soon I got tired of this, and started giving answers such as: "I am in a horse barn, and the President of the United States is George Washington!" Adelle, one of my favorite nurses said, "If you continue to give sassy answers like that, you will *never* leave the hospital!"

One thing I did not look forward to was "belly shots" of heparin in the morning and at night to prevent blood clots. Pretty soon I was ranking the nurses from 1-10, which made them nervous. I thought when I was transferred to rehabilitation in-between treatments, maybe they did not do that, but I was not so lucky! In the beginning, I had to wear those white stockings, but I quit that when I started to become more active.

Thursday, November 19

Today is my mom's birthday. She is 84 years old. Transferred to Mass Eye and Ear Spaulding Rehabilitation. Intensive rehabilitation, physical and occupational therapy. Started wearing real clothes, like sweats and shirts, and never went back to johnnies again! The menu here was excellent. Besides, you could order anything you wanted from the kitchen all day. Spring water, as many bottles as you wished, tall bottles of Tropicana orange juice, not those little plastic containers that took two swallows. There was only one floor there for rehab patients, so service was more accommodating than usual.

Saturday, November 20

Georgia's husband, Ron, arrived to be with her and to have Thanksgiving with her. Their kids, Nicole, Michelle, and Michael, encouraged their dad to be with their mom, that they would be just fine having Thanksgiving themselves.

Sunday, November 21

My birthday. My room was totally filled with friends, family, flowers and gifts, including lots of stuffed animals and chocolate and laughter. Most of these friends supported me when I had cancer twelve years ago. Some were friends for over 20 years. Most didn't just come once; they carpooled and came several times. I am so blessed!

My mom knew where I was as I moved here and there. Georgia kept her informed, and I talked to my mom every day. I felt she was with me.

Monday, November 22

Portacath with two entry ports put into chest. (one port for chemotherapy or hydration, and the other to draw blood at the same time.)

Georgia was getting anxious waiting for me because it was taking longer than they originally told her. So, another incident that was added to my major problems was: When the doctors were putting the portacath into my chest, they punctured my lung (pneumo-thorax) by mistake. They had to put a tube into my chest wall to correct the situation. Every day I had to have an X-ray to see how the lung was filling up. They brought the X-ray equipment to my bed. The two main doctors and a colleague came into my room every day. I could see by their faces how truly sorry they were.

Recovery from that was the most severe pain I ever had in the hospital, more than any test or procedure. I self-administered morphine with a button that was attached to my IV line. You know that paper where you practically sign your life away? The doctor said that this happens to one percent of people. I guess I very neatly fit into that category!

Remember, I was also dealing with a left fractured clavicle and recovering from eye surgery at the time.

When my lung recovered, it was time to take the tube out of my chest wall. Dr. Cook asked me to take three deep breaths in and out. On the third exhalation, he quickly pulled the tube from my chest wall. I did not know he was going to remove the tube, so when I took that deep breath, I did not feel the tube come out. It was bloody, but I wanted to take it back on the plane with me to show my mom. He said it might be a health hazard, and he would bring an unused one, but I never saw him again.

Monday, November 26

Chemo cycle #2. Did not get sick. MRI after this showed shrinkage of tumors.

Monday, November 29

Transferred to rehabilitation at Mass Eye and Ear Spaulding. Intensive rehabilitation.

Tuesday, November 30

Ron said goodbye and went back home to California. MRI 10:p.m.

Monday, December 6

Chemo cycle #3. Did not get sick.

Thursday, December 9

Georgia left to go back to California. (Note: Later Georgia told me the nurses encouraged her to wean herself away from me, leaving me alone longer every day.) She had been through the roughest times with me. It was a sad parting for both of us. She felt she had "brought me along," and now she was leaving unfinished business. I felt like a child whose mother had gone away. In some ways, it was like déja vu 12 years ago when my mother had to leave me in Massachusetts and return to her home in California, after months of taking care of me, my two sons and my dog. (I still don't know how she did it.) What a horrible lonely, abandoned feeling!

Transferred to Mass General Hospital Spaulding Rehabilitation. Many patients, all floors here. More chaos than the rehab at Mass Eyeand Ear. Wherever there was a bed open, that is where they took me. I had no choice.

Monday, December 20

Chemo cycle #4. Did not get sick. MRI showed tumors completely gone!!! Dr. Hochberg said that when my tumors were gone, I only had to do two more cycles. Hallelujah!!! After cycle #4, I was not eligible to go to rehab, so I went to live in the apartment Georgia had rented, foreseeing this possibility. I had a visiting nurse and physical or occupational therapist come at one time to evaluate me, but I didn't need help then, or even later.

Picture this. There was a step to the main entrance to the building. Inside the door, where the mailboxes were, there were no handrails, so I had to crawl up the steps. My apartment was in the basement, so I had to go down tons of steps. The hand railing didn't start at the top of the steps, so I went down on my butt until I could reach for the handrail.

There was a sliding door off the kitchen that led out to the alley with a lot of trash cans. It was kind of narrow and uneven for walking. One advantage was that it was only a few steps down from the sidewalk. Because the alley was harder for walking, I opted for the front entrance. Can you imagine if I fell in the alley and nobody found me for days? Now *that* would have been sad and very pathetic!

Tuesday, December 21

Radiation #1—the molded mask is fit snugly over my face, nose, and chin. After they clamp it down, one side is radiated, and then the other. The whole radiation process takes a couple minutes, but the real pain in the neck was waiting for up to an hour for transport to take me back to my room. As the minutes passed, I told the man at the desk to call transport again. Finally I said, "If someone doesn't come pretty soon, I am going to cry!" By now, I was feeling very frustrated and abandoned, so that was not just a threat. I am prone to tears easily. I know the staff is busy, as I saw other patients being parked in some space, waiting, waiting, waiting, and sensed that the other patients were also feeling tired and forgotten. Here again, if you are a patient in a hospital, you have no control. Being so dependent on people was the main motivation that empowered me to strive *intensely* to get well!

Wednesday, December 22

Radiation #2

Thursday, December 23

Radiation #3

Friday, December 24

Approximately on this date, a father and his son delivered Christmas cards the son had made for the patients. I was touched. Two or three Salvation Army men stood outside my room, with Christmas music coming out of their horns. I put the Santa hat that Georgia bought for me on my stuffed elephant from David and Gina. (Too many stuffed animals in my room, so some were taken to the apartment. Before I went home, I paid over $100 to ship everything to California.) What a blessed Christmas—not quite like home, but I felt the Spirit.

Monday, December 27

Radiation #4

Tuesday, December 28

Radiation #5

Wednesday, December 29

Radiation #6

Thursday, December 30

Radiation #7

Saturday, January 1, 2000

New Year's Day. Home nurse and home aide visit at my apartment to evaluate me to see if I would need help. I was fine as I demonstrated to them my ability to be independent. I never saw them again.

Monday, January 3

Radiation #8

Tuesday, January 4

Radiation #9 and Chemo cycle #5

Wednesday, January 5

Radiation #10—Last one.

Thursday, January 7

Back to the apartment. Gave me a chance to see my friends in a non-hospital environment. We even walked down the street to what got to be my favorite restaurant, The Phoenicia. Lebanese food, yummy! Hummus, kibbee, lamb shish-ka-bob, tabouleh, baklava, etc. More than one of my friends got addicted to this fantastic savoring food. What a wonderful thing I was experiencing! (When Georgia brought this food to me in the hospital many times, the hospital food on my tray never got touched.)

Tuesday, January 18

Chemo cycle #6—Last one. Hallelujah!!!! Glory be to God! I got sick the last fifteen minutes of Methotrexate. But, hey, it's the last chemo treatment, so what the heck?!

Wednesday, January 26

Farewell Massachusetts. Hello sunny California and home sweet home. I had mixed emotions, as I was leaving my long-time friends, my doctors and nurses who did so much for me, and all of whom I got attached, or reattached. Of course, they were all glad I was getting better, but no one wanted to see me go. On the other hand, I had family and friends eagerly waiting for me to return. What a wonderful blessing to have friends and family who love me from coast to coast. Thank you God for everything!

To divert slightly:
Rehabilitation process at home in California
I started with the walker. But, I was the one who told physical therapy I was ready for a four-pronged cane, and I was the one who decided when to transfer to a regular cane. I finally stopped using the cane, against my doctors' and nurses' wishes. I felt that it was becoming a burden instead of a crutch or help.

When it was time to drive alone, I decided to drive to my mom's house in the same village. As I was backing out of the garage, I was so excited. I said to myself, "Oh, my God, I can't believe I am actually driving!"

This attitude continued as I got tired of depending on people to drive me everywhere, so when I got a prism in my glasses to prevent double vision, I took driver training to get my confidence back.

================================

The following two-page article appeared in April 20, 2000 issue of the Massachusetts General Hospital newsletter, called "Caring Headlines, Occupational Therapy Month":
Exemplar
Occupational therapy helps patient regain functional abilities, self-esteem. My name is Kathy Wilcox and I have been an occupational therapist for seven and a half years, most recently, at MGH for one year. I was originally drawn to OT by the profession's unique approach to helping people regain functional independence using everyday activities. My special interest is working with neuro patients.

I first met Diane Jepsen in October, 1999, when she was admitted for a treatment for a central nervous system ocular lymphoma that attacked her for the second time in 12 years. She was lying in bed as her sister fed her from a bedside table. My first thought was how humbling it must be to be fed by someone else. Diane shared these same feelings with me during our first meeting. I soon discovered Diane had difficulty feeding herself due to arm tremors, trunk and extremity weakness and double vision. The cancer had invaded her cerebellum and her right eye (primary targets). {Note from Diane: Both eyes had lymphoma, but the biopsy was done in the right eye.}

I introduced myself and explained the role of occupational therapy. I set out to adapt her environment to promote independence for her. The first step was to set her up in bed as she wasn't able to get into a chair or support herself while sitting on the edge of the bed. Once this was accomplished with help from me and her nurse, I lowered the bedside table to a level where she could rest her elbows comfortably. I showed Diane how to position her elbows to provide proximal arm stability to minimize the ataxia (tremors) that occurred with any movement, especially in her dominant right hand.

Once in this position, Diane was able to grasp utensils and feed herself most of the solid foods that had been pre-cut for her. A long straw was provided to alleviate holding a cup and risk spilling, due to her tremors. I put a patch on her right eye to eliminate the double vision. I instructed both Diane and her sister in these activities, which gave Diane a sense of control and independence. They were then able to instruct other staff on how to re-create this set-up for future meals and continue to promote self-reliance. They were both very excited! Diane expressed a sense of relief and optimism.

The next day I met with Diane to establish additional functional goals. First, we identified the barriers to her participation in self-care. She had impairments in dynamic sitting balance, mobility, fine and gross motor coordination, proprioception (position sense), overall strength, vision, short-term memory and impulse control. {Note from Diane: Was I a mess or what?}

Next, we collaborated on prioritizing the goals that were important to Diane. These included feeding herself, transferring to a commode and ultimately to a toilet, performing her own grooming tasks, and walking to the bathroom to take a shower. Most of us forget how important these "simple" tasks are to our self-esteem.

Diane approached therapy the same way she approached life, full of optimism, spirit, and always with humor and a sniffle. I was amazed at her positive attitude. This played a major role in her recovery. Divorced for 23 years, she was a very independent woman. She had been diagnosed and successfully treated for lymphoma at MGH 12 years earlier. She had then moved to California to be near her mother and sister. There she worked part-time as a receptionist, and created a newsletter for her neighborhood community {Note from Diane: This was actually in Acton, Massachusetts in 1990, years *before* I moved to California.} She also practiced yoga regularly.

Knowing her desire to be productive and active, it was important that we established realistic goals in this early phase while she was undergoing chemotherapy. Her sister played a vital role in helping Diane to carry over the functional techniques we worked on together. Our therapy began with the 'simple' task of sitting on the edge of the bed and completing the functional goal of brushing her teeth. This was challenging because of the ataxia in her torso. Our goal was for Diane to brush her teeth without assistance, while maintaining her sitting balance on the edge of the bed.

(Note from Diane: I don't ever remember not being able to brush my teeth, but Georgia told me that initially she had to do that for me.)

She then progressed from transfers from a bed to a chair, walking [with a walker] from the bed to a chair in front of the bathroom sink, and finally walking [with a walker] to the bathroom to stand at the sink. Once she was able to stand at the sink, she could brush her teeth independently. Between chemotherapy cycles, Diane would go to a rehabilitation facility, returning for her cycle, stronger and more determined. The final challenge came during her third chemotherapy cycle: taking a shower. By this time, she was using a walker with supervision to walk. I set up a shower chair and instructed Diane how to safely transfer into the shower using the grab bars and her walker. She was able to complete her shower by using the hand-held shower with supervision and an occasional safety instruction. She had achieved her goal.

I did not need to see Diane when she returned from her final three chemo cycles. She had been discharged from the rehabilitation facility, and was living independently in a Boston apartment. Her sister had returned to California. Diane was able to prepare a light meal in the kitchen without assistance, using only a straight cane for support.

I asked Diane how she viewed her experience with occupational therapy. This is what she told me; "(It) has been very exciting. I have learned to master kitchen skills, as well as showering, dressing and feeding myself. (OT) was key in helping me return to independent living while regaining the self-esteem that slipped away when my illness set in."

Diane returned to her home in California at the end of January, with a clean bill of health, having regained independence and self-confidence about taking care of herself at home. It was a bittersweet goodbye for both of us; we had become accustomed to our visits. It was then that I realized the impact we had had on each other.

Comments by Jeanette Ives Erickson, RN, MS, senior vice-president for Patient Care and chief nurse

Kathy's narrative eloquently describes the work of the occupational therapist. She is able to alter this patient's environment to allow for the highest level of independent functioning. Diane's life has been profoundly changed by her illness—her future is uncertain. You can imagine the fear and anxiety she felt. {Note from Diane: I was anxious at times, but I was never afraid.}

Using her extensive knowledge and expertise, Kathy helps Diane regain control of her life. Together, they identify goals and priorities and work diligently to overcome the limitations brought on by Diane's illness. Kathy's creativity, resourcefulness, skill and compassion are evident throughout this entire narrative. Thank you, Kathy

======================

Since I have returned to California, I have been having "maintenance/preventive chemotherapy" which has been scheduled for once a month for three months, and then every three months, three times. My oncologist here, Dr. Warren Paroly, is a knowledgeable and compassionate doctor, with a sense of humor who has followed Dr. Hochberg's protocol for treatment to the nth degree. He said, "Why mess with a good thing?" Dr. Paroly has an equally compassionate assistant named Chris Lewis, who taught me about spiral meditation and mind-body-touch healing. There is also a trained staff of oncology nurses (one of my favorites is Cher) at Tri-City Hospital in Oceanside, CA which makes me feel secure. I continue with MRI (To date I have had twenty!) and lumbar puncture (drawing fluid from the spine) to check for cancer cells in the body. They won't find anything.

Note: On Sunday, September 3, approximately midnight, this thought came to me: Would more chemo be harmful instead of helpful to me? The very next day, I sent a detailed letter to my doctors stating this concern. Today is November 11, and I have not had a response except on my answering machine that one of my doctors was on vacation (which is hardly a response). I am scheduled for chemo Tuesday, November 14, and temporarily again in February 2001. That is not going to happen, as long as the doctors don't inform me why the chemos were scheduled as they were. After my tumors were gone after chemo #4 in Massachusetts, I was administered two more treatments. In addition, I have had five "maintenance chemo" treatments in California after that. What would two more chemos do? Ten more chemos? One hundred more chemos? Or NO more chemos?

If there is no answer, then I will make the decision to go on with my life and activities with energy and passion. Not even to look back, and not be worried about this and that. There are too many unknowns that we all deal with every day, so why worry?

OK, here is an update:

After calling Dr. Paroly's office, I called the hospital and canceled my chemo that was scheduled for November 14. I did go to the lab, and also saw Dr. Paroly on November 13. Upon entering the examining room, he said "You just can't stay away from us, can you?" He sat down and said, "You are not going to like what you are going to hear. Dr. Hochberg thinks you need to have chemo every three months the rest of your life because of your unusual cancer that recurs."

I told him I thought that was too aggressive since there was no proof on which to base the frequency decision. He said that Dr. Hochberg was the expert. I am not so stupid as to reject treatment, especially since Dr. Hochberg was key in saving my life twice. Dr. Paroly wanted me to schedule my own appointment, which I did for January 23, 2001. When I said, "How about six months?" he said, "Why don't we talk after your chemo?" That really took the weight off.

As Georgia remembered Dr. Sang saying, the victrectomy (eye biopsy) would cause a cataract in my right eye. At the initial appointment before surgery here, the eye surgeon agreed that this was a typical victrectomy cataract. Surgery will probably be done in February.

33.

SOME POSITIVE THOUGHTS

- While in Massachusetts for second cancer August 1999 to January 2000, I was able to see my two sons, Peter, 29, New York, and David, 26, Boston.
- I had the honor to meet, know and love Gina, who asked me to look at wedding dresses with her (before I got *really* sick).
- David and Gina lived very close to the hospital, and she is a top-of-the-line nurse in cardiac care at Massachusetts General Hospital. I was truly lucky, as they were nearby, and so were able to visit and help me. David kept Peter informed, so I had visits and regular phone calls from him.
- I actually enjoyed my time there, and saw many nurses and therapists again and again, as I went back and forth to the hospital and rehabilitation. Relationships were formed. One therapist wrote on my form next to the word safety: "Impulsive". (Sometimes I took leaps when they thought I wasn't ready.)
- I enjoyed all my roommates. I even saw some more than once. Each had a story to tell:

–One was run over by a trolley.

–Another was in a house fire where she lost two children. Her husband threw her out the window to save her, and now she has only one leg.

–Another woman's marriage became more solid, as her husband had to take care of the kids. She vowed not to be so picky, and little things about how the kids looked when they came to visit, didn't bother her anymore. Like maybe the kids were not as clean, or they had their shirts inside out.

–There was another woman who wore earrings and makeup and a white bow in her hair. I did not know what ailed her, but she certainly did not look sick. I do know that she had not been able to eat for days, maybe 30. I encouraged her to at least try to eat some mashed potatoes. She was able to do that, and she was proud of herself. I was proud of her, too!

–Let us not forget Mary, an elderly woman, who told me that she didn't want the male aide who was taking care of her, to think that he was her boyfriend. She was connected to her oxygen in the wall, but when she was in the wheelchair, she wheeled herself to the door, because she wanted to go home. She stretched her oxygen cord to the extent that she almost pulled it out of the wall. This worried me, and I was constantly calling the nurses. She said, "I am going to call the cops so they can take me home, but I will let you talk, because you can talk better than I can." More than once she asked, "Is your husband with Ralph?" I said, "I don't have a husband, and I don't know who Ralph is."

–There was a woman who couldn't speak English, so her husband stayed with her day and night to interpret questions from nurses and doctors. I always saw him in the same sweater. I think she had some sort of brain tumor, and her doctors did not give her a good prognosis. I am glad I was there for him so that we could talk together. I remember he always had on the same s sweater. Never left to change his clothes.

Many, many more stories. I told the nurses that everyone around me seemed to be sicker than I was. They said, "You should have seen yourself when you first came in!"

Medically, I was not supposed to live, but I did. Whenever I saw Dr. Hochberg's face, I was lifted. When he visited my bed, I always tried to perform at my very best, because like a little girl seeking approval, I wanted him to be proud of me. A couple days before I left the hospital, I thanked him and said, "Well, we did it again—that's two times now!" He said, "So far." Pointing to him, I shot back, "So far for you, too!"

Actually, all of us who are living on this earth are in the "so-far" stage. So, live life to the fullest every day, be kind to one another, but most of all, don't let the devil get you!

I am not living by accident, but as a result of many blessings to me from the love and grace of God. If you add to this, great family and friends and doctors and nurses, you can't get any better than this! I am now improving and growing stronger every day in every way—spiritually, mentally and physically.

Finally a big THANK YOU to my mom who called me every day from California, wishing she could be with me, tracking me down as I got moved to and fro. She was and is such an inspiration to me. I wrote this poem on my bed while at Emerson Hospital in Concord, Massachusetts:

My Mother

Mothers are mothers,
They come and they go
From the top of the mountains
To the valleys below.
They soothe your tears and nurture your soul;
They lift you up when you're feeling low;
They get down on their knees to pray
That God will show them the way.

Mine is special—I'll tell you why;
When my face flows with tears
She wipes them dry
With a loving hand and an understanding eye.

She's beautiful and loving and secure and strong,
And *always* admits when she is wrong!!!!????
She's the one you want next to your bed,
Or cheering you on in your moment of dread.

She has touched and enriched others far and wide;
You would always want her to be on your side;
She's one in a million sent from heaven above,
To give all her children everlasting love.

So, God bless my mother on this special day,
And may His Spirit enfold her in every way.

Love,
Diane

Addendum

Sunrise, Sunset— Quickly go the Years

Since I have returned to California in January 2000, much has happened. It is impossible for me to recall everything, but I would like to give my readers some updates, and also share some new developments.

- Maintenance chemotherapy treatments were initiated in California, beginning February 22, 2000, and continued every month for three months; then treatment was scheduled once every three months. When doctors couldn't tell me whether too much chemo was more harmful than helpful, I decided to gradually lengthen the frequency of my treatments. There was no opposition to my decision; in fact, I was given control over setting up my own lab dates and chemo appointments at the hospital.
- My last treatment was October 7, 2003. I got very sick with nausea and vomiting on multiple times. Phlegm came out of my mouth and nose, and I was shaking and crying. I said to myself, "Forget about moving the frequency up to six months. I will not do this for another year." My thoughts kept moving along as I was lying in my bed thinking, and I said to myself, "That's it. I quit chemo now!"
- My cancer was gone in December 1999; then I was given two more treatments, just to make sure. If I have to have chemo the rest of my life, then

the reasoning should be: *Everyone* (Just exaggerating, but you get my point!) should have chemo in the event one tiny cancer cell might be hiding. My California oncologist, Dr. Paroly, and I made a deal: Twice a year I would have MRIs, lab work, and also office appointments with him. My last MRI (No.27) was October 11, 2005.

- My portocath was surgically removed April 29, 2004. I am going to die one day, but I truly believe it will not be due to cancer.
- I make annual "hug" trips back to see Dr. Fred Hocherg at Massachusetts General Hospital in Boston. These are unbelievable reunions, and he is always calling other doctors or interns in to meet me, and saying something such as, "This is the woman I was telling you about" or "Doctors will learn more from Diane Jepsen than they will in school."
- My younger son, David, was married to Kristin, June 14, 2003, and now I am a first-time grandmother with a beautiful granddaughter, Caroline Elisabeth, who was born May 20, 2004.
- My older son, Peter, continues to thrive, living and working in New York, as a portfolio manager, trading currency. He recently became engaged to Brooke; the wedding date is planned for October 2006.
- Two spectacular women—what mothers pray and hope for their sons!
- My mother, 90, and her husband, Muxie, 92, recently celebrated their tenth wedding anniversary. They live only four blocks from my home.
- My sister, Georgia, and husband, Ron, come to visit often and are always available to help in every way.
- I continue to improve: I was told that if I did not have double vision, I would not need glasses.
- I drive almost everywhere I need to go, but *not* the freeways! When I told Dr. Hochberg this on one of my "hug" visits, he said, "That's because you're smart!"
- My walking and strength continues to improve, as I work out in the fitness here in my village. At this writing, I am able to leg press over 130 lbs.
- I know I am unable to do some things because I am aware of my limitations. However, if I try, voila! I can do something I never thought I could ever do.
- I wash my own car, clean my own house, and basically take care of my entire patio.
- I sing in my church choir, and have compiled poems from choir members to produce a book with my friend, Jim, called *Poetry from the Choir Loft.*

- I have become more and more knowledgeable with the computer, including custom-designing greeting cards to send to family and friends.
- The total experience of cancer, not once, but twice, has been a gift to me. My faith in God has increased one-hundred-fold. I know that He loves me and will care for me every day. Either He will shield me from suffering or He will give me unfailing strength to bear it. Because of this faith, I put aside all anxious thoughts and fears. What, me worry? Give it to God. Let Him do it!

"Who comforteth us in all our tribulation that we may be able to comfort them which are in any trouble, by the comfort wherewith we ourselves are comforted of God."

II Corinthians 1:4

Sunrise, sunset, quickly go the years.

* * * * *

EPILOGUE

by Georgia Tamoush

To put into words what Diane went through, what we went through together is nearly impossible. Diane is so feisty, strong-willed and determined. I can still hear her response to Dr. Hochberg, when he said to her, "You could die." She said. "You could die, too!"

This is one extraordinary person who taught me a lot during our weeks together. Even with five brain tumors, lymphoma in both eyes, a broken clavicle, and a punctured lung, with all the pain she endured, Diane's sense of humor never waned. She joked with every doctor, every nurse, every staff member, and lifted the spirits of all the patients. Diane is an inspiration to me and to many whose paths she crossed during her ordeal. I am so thankful that I had the opportunity to be with her in Boston. I will never forget our tough fight together, the love we shared, and her unbelievable and unmatched courage.

About the Author

Diane Fadel Jepsen thinks of herself as the "chosen one," as she is a survivor of brain cancer, not once, but twice. She sees cancer as a "gift," which has enriched her faith and ways of spirituality. She has a greater understanding and sensitivity to others' challenges and limitations, and what really matters in life. Diane's wish is to be God's instrument of hope in other people's lives.

"I think I can, I think I can, I think I can."
—*The Little Engine That Could,* Watty Piper, 1930

Contacting the Author

Diane Fadel Jepsen
4739 Majorca Way
Oceanside, CA 92056-5118
dfjepsen@cox.com

Publisher:
www.iuniverse.com
402-323-7800

978-0-595-21880-6
0-595-21880-6

LaVergne, TN USA
17 September 2009
158181LV00001B/226/A